Surgical Care in the
United States

The Johns Hopkins Series in Contemporary Medicine and Public Health

Consulting editors:
Martin D. Abeloff, M.D.
Samuel H. Boyer, M.D.
Gareth M. Green, M.D.
Richard T. Johnson, M.D.
Paul R. McHugh, M.D.
Edmond A. Murphy, M.D.
Edyth H. Schoenrich, M.D., M.P.H.
Jerry L. Spivak, M.D.
Barbara H. Starfield, M.D., M.P.H.

Also of interest in this series:

Hospital Structure and Performance, Ann Barry Flood and W. Richard Scott

Medicaid and Pediatric Primary Care, Janet D. Perloff, Phillip R. Kletke, and Kathryn M. Neckerman

Uncompensated Hospital Care: Rights and Responsibilities, Frank A. Sloan, James F. Blumstein, and James M. Perrin, eds.

The Effectiveness of Medical Care: Validating Clinical Wisdom, Barbara H. Starfield and others

The Hospital Power Equilibrium: Physician Behavior and Cost Control, David W. Young and Richard B. Saltman

Surgical Care in the United States
A Policy Perspective

edited by

Madelon Lubin Finkel
*Clinical Associate Professor of Public Health
Cornell University Medical College*

The Johns Hopkins University Press
Baltimore and London

© 1988 The Johns Hopkins University Press
All rights reserved
Printed in the United States of America

The Johns Hopkins University Press, 701 West 40th Street,
Baltimore, Maryland 21211
The Johns Hopkins Press Ltd., London

The paper used in this publication meets the minimum requirements of
American National Standard for Information Sciences—Permanence of Paper
for Printed Library Materials, ANSI Z39.48-1984.

Library of Congress Cataloging-in Publication Data
Surgical care in the United States : a policy perspective / edited by
   Madelon Lubin Finkel.
       p. cm.—(The Johns Hopkins series in contemporary medicine
   and public health)
   Includes bibliographies and index.
   ISBN 0-8018-3638-7 (alk. paper)
   1. Surgery—Economic aspects—United States.   2. Surgery—
Government policy—United States.   I. Finkel, Madelon Lubin, 1949–.   II.
Series.
   [DNLM: 1. Delivery of Health Care—United States.   2. Health Policy—
economics—United States.   3. Surgery—United States.   WO 100 S9622]
   RD27.42.S87   1988
   362.1'97—dc19
   DNLM/DLC
   for Library of Congress   88-606
                                                                              CIP

Contents

Contributors   vii
Introduction   1

1. Surgical Care in Developed Nations
   Eugene Vayda and Janet M. Barnsley   11
2. Surgical Operations and Manpower Considerations
   Ira M. Rutkow   22
3. Regional Variation in Surgical Procedures
   Madelon Lubin Finkel   41
4. Variation in Surgical Practice: A Proposal for Action
   John Wennberg   58
5. The Evaluation of Surgical Care
   Francis D. Moore   80
6. Managing Surgical Admissions
   Leslie L. Roos and Noralou P. Roos   107
7. Surgery and the Changing System of Health Care Delivery
   Dan Ermann   125
8. Identifying Hospitals for the Regionalization of Care
   Harold S. Luft and Sandra S. Hunt   144
9. The Federal Assessment of Surgical Procedures
   Jane E. Sisk and Gloria Ruby   159
10. What Does the Future Hold?
    Leslie L. Roos   175

Index   191

Contributors

Janet M. Barnsley, M.S., Department of Health Administration, Division of Community Health, Faculty of Medicine, University of Toronto

Dan Ermann, M.B.A., M.P.H., National Center for Health Services Research and Health Care Technology Assessment, U.S. Department of Health and Human Services

Sandra S. Hunt, M.P.A., Institute for Health Policy Studies, School of Medicine, University of California, San Francisco

Harold S. Luft, Ph.D., Institute for Health Policy Studies, School of Medicine, University of California, San Francisco

Francis D. Moore, M.D., Moseley Professor of Surgery Emeritus, Harvard Medical School; president, Massachusetts Health Data Consortium, Inc. (1981–1986); editorial staff, *New England Journal of Medicine*

Leslie L. Roos, Ph.D., Professor of Management and Medicine, University of Manitoba; National Health Scientists, Government of Canada

Noralou P. Roos, Ph.D., Professor of Management and Medicine, University of Manitoba; National Health Scientists, Government of Canada

Gloria Ruby, M.A., Senior Analyst, Health Program, Office of Technology Assessment, U.S. Congress

Ira M. Rutkow, M.D., M.P.H., Dr.P.H., Freehold Area Hospital, Freehold, N.J.

Jane E. Sisk, Ph.D., Senior Associate, Health Program, Office of Technology Assessment, U.S. Congress

Eugene Vayda, M.D., Department of Health Administration, Division of Community Health, Faculty of Medicine, University of Toronto

John Wennberg, M.D., Professor of Epidemiology, Department of Community and Family Medicine, Dartmouth Medical School

Surgical Care in the
United States

Introduction

Advances in the biomedical sciences and the development of sophisticated medical technology have all but eliminated many of the illnesses and diseases that used to cripple and kill. The life expectancy for all cultural groups has increased, and statistics indicate that, as a nation, we are growing healthier. At the same time, requests for medical care and the costs of such care have skyrocketed. Neither the federal budget nor the national debt has increased as rapidly as health care costs. The quality of medical care and the access to that care could be jeopardized by economics.

The utilization and financing of medical care in the United States have undergone rapid changes in the past two decades, with more change during the last few years than during the preceding twenty years. In the past, physicians exercised broad discretionary powers in organizing their practices and in managing patients: they would decide on the number and type of tests to order, when to hospitalize, and when to discharge. Now outside forces increasingly dictate the patterns of medical practice.

The health maintenance organization, the preferred provider organization, and for-profit, multihospital systems have altered the way in which health care is delivered and paid for, while consumer concerns about the high cost of health care have spurred the implementation of various cost-management programs, such as preadmission certification, mandatory second opinions, home health care, ambulatory surgical centers, and managed care. Managed care, the newest concept in the delivery of health care, is designed to establish standards that physicians must follow in an attempt to control "unnecessary" and costly interventions. Advances in medical technology, new methods of financing (diagnosis-related groups, prospective rate setting), and new delivery systems (walk-in clinics, ambulatory surgical centers) have revolutionized health care.

Employers are becoming informed and prudent purchasers of health care rather than mere payers of claims. In addition, they are redesigning health benefit plans to include incentives for employees to seek cost-effective care. Improvements in the available information on the utilization, cost, and quality of health care enable purchasers to channel patients toward "efficient" providers; that is, employers and insurers are now able to identify cost-efficient providers and can exercise their purchasing power to reward such hospitals and physicians with more patients. The aim is to contain costs while encouraging the appropriate use of medical facilities and personnel. What effect these measures have on the quality of care is yet to be quantified, however.

The established system has been significantly changed by the rapid increase in entrepreneurial activities by both for-profit and nonprofit health care organizations as well as by the increasingly successful efforts of the business sector to renegotiate benefit plans to encourage employees to enroll in alternatives to traditional fee-for-service arrangements. Competition has accelerated the trend toward group practice and salaried positions for physicians. The destabilization is further exacerbated by the growing excess of hospital beds and physicians.

The rise in the number of physicians has far-reaching implications for the health care system. Stimulated by predictions in the 1960s that there would be too few physicians to meet the needs of the expanding population, new medical schools were established and existing ones expanded their enrollment. Between 1960 and 1985, the number of new physicians doubled. The number of physicians per 100,000 people is estimated to increase significantly by the end of the century, and this increase will create a tougher, more competitive environment for physicians, particularly for younger, well-trained physicians. Most physicians in the 1980s are working shorter hours than their colleagues did in the 1950s and 1960s, and per capita visits to physicians have been declining rapidly over the past decade, further complicating the situation.

Young resident physicians in almost all medical subspecialties are finding that many fields are already saturated, that competition for patients is keen, and that many community hospitals are unwilling to accept additional doctors on staff. Physicians have moved into smaller, previously underserved communities, and this process of geographic diffusion has led to a wider availability of specialized services in rural areas.

Given the new climate of cost consciousness and an increased supply of physicians, it is not surprising that the provision of medical care has come under the scrutiny of policy researchers. The rapid changes that have occurred present a variety of challenges to the medical profession. It appears to many that the goal of public policy has shifted away from ensuring access to care toward controlling the rising cost of care.

Hospital services are the most frequent target for the management of health care costs. Hospitalization is the most expensive aspect of health care, and within this category, surgery is the most costly component. Thus, it is argued, any program that reduces hospital stay in general and surgical care in particular is almost certain to save money.

Researchers have realized that an undetermined proportion of surgical procedures may be unnecessary. The likelihood of an individual's undergoing elective surgery has increased dramatically over the last fifteen years. It is estimated that at least one-third of the hysterectomies and two-thirds of the tonsillectomies performed need not have been. Unnecessary surgery also has been reported for ophthalmologic and orthopedic procedures. The increasing rates of surgery, their concomitant costs, and the possibility that some procedures are performed without medical justification has provided the impetus for second surgical opinion programs.

This volume focuses on the surgical profession in examining changes that have occurred in the delivery of health care in the United States in the post–Medicare/Medicaid decades. Many of the chapters are the products of years of research and provide up-to-date accounts of topics that directly affect the provision of health care and surgical care. These chapters illustrate problems that the surgical community must address as we approach the twenty-first century.

NATIONAL AND INTERNATIONAL VARIATION IN SURGICAL CARE

Persistent questions about the cost and medical appropriateness of surgery have given rise to several approaches to studying and controlling the levels of utilization of surgical care. One issue that has generated considerable debate is whether the surgery being performed in the United States is excessive. Although the evidence is not conclusive, findings from numerous studies conducted over the past fifteen years clearly show that the geographic variation in the number of surgical procedures performed is more than one would expect by chance alone. These differences indicate that the frequency of surgical intervention in some areas may be inappropriate. But do lower numbers of procedures imply simply that too little surgery is being performed? Do higher numbers imply that too much surgery is being performed?

Elective surgery inherently involves a wide range of factors related to, among other things, the patient's perception of disability and the surgeon's estimation of the potential benefit of the operation. It is well known that surgeons' evaluations of the need for surgical intervention vary widely. In second-opinion programs, the rates of nonconfirmation of proposed surgical procedures vary from less than 5 percent to over 40 percent. Orthopedic and gynecologic procedures show the highest variation, whereas general surgical procedures show the least variation.

Studies have shown that the degree of variation generally appears to be characteristic of the specific procedure more than of the geographic area in which it was performed. Differences of opinion appear to influence practice patterns similarly in the United States and abroad. The procedures with little variation seem to be those for which there is a consensus among surgeons concerning appropriate treatment. However, other interventions—for example, the use of hysterectomy for non-cancerous conditions—are a continuing source of professional controversy. The use of cholecystectomy, too, varies primarily because of differing attitudes toward the removal of asymptomatic gallstones.

These differences raise a set of difficult questions about the quality and cost efficiency of surgical care in the United States. The number of physicians poses another set of questions: Are we producing "too many" highly trained surgeons for the needs of the population? Are specific subspecialties more glutted than others? Do previously underserved geographic regions now have "enough" physicians and surgeons for the needs of the population?

Chapter 1, citing national and regional data, compares the utilizations of surgical care in developed nations. Cross-national studies highlight the differences in the numbers of surgical procedures performed and raise anew the issue of the necessity of surgery. The cross-national differences continue to be a subject of concern, and Dr. Vayda and Ms. Barnsley focus on possible explanations for the wide variations. Confounding the issue, however, is the lack of consensus on optimal levels of surgery for particular diagnoses. Efforts are under way to identify a research agenda regarding the efficacy of surgical treatments and the modification of physicians' behaviors based on regional and small-area comparisons.

Chapter 2, which examines surgical operations and the growth of the surgical profession, provides an overview of the most frequently performed operations in eight surgical subspecialties. Data clearly show the increases that have occurred in these interventions, as well as the increase in the number of surgeons during the same period. Dr. Rutkow concludes that the United States faces a glut of surgeons of unprecedented proportion that has significant implications for surgeons and patients alike. Studies show that fewer operations are being performed, making it difficult for surgeons to maintain their technical skills. The indications for operations may become less stringent, which may result in "unnecessary" surgery. Dr. Rutkow calls for surgeons to evaluate the situation and take steps to confront the problem in the immediate future.

Chapter 3 focuses on regional variation in surgical care. Accepting the premise that variation exists and that its explanations are often not well understood, I cite trends in the procedure-specific utilization of surgery over a decade in four geographic areas. In some cases, the regional differences are substantial, as are the costs associated with the surgical procedure. The explanations for the increases are not obvious. It is clear that individual surgical subspecialties must be analyzed before generalizations can be made about the extent of unnecessary surgery being performed in some areas.

VARIATION IN SURGICAL CARE WITHIN SMALL AREAS

In recent years, researchers and policymakers have focused their attention on variations in surgical care across geographic areas, and in particular across small areas. These studies have attracted the attention of insurers and government as they seek to contain medical expenditures by choosing providers and systems of medical care. Different practice patterns, different practice settings, and different criteria for surgery or diagnostic testing contribute to variations in surgical care within and between areas. The extent to which these variations compromise patient care is not known.

Analysis of data from small areas is an excellent means of investigating the differences in clinical decision making because the number of surgical procedures performed in a specific area is a direct consequence of decisions made by a small group of physicians. The evidence suggests that variations occur primarily in those "gray areas" in which presumably equally competent physicians disagree on the preferred course of treatment. The practice styles of individual surgeons emerge as important factors in understanding different patterns of surgery.

Policymakers are trying to reduce or manage costs while assuring the quality of care. Because small-area analysis may prove useful in cost containment, it has drawn the interest of government policymakers. The savings in reimbursement costs could be substantial if the high rates of surgery in one area could be brought into line with the lower rates found in a neighboring area. Conversely, population-based data are also important in identifying areas of low use where lack of access to surgical care should be studied.

Dr. Wennberg's work on variation among small areas has contributed significantly to our understanding of the relationship between clinical medicine and the economics, politics, and regulation of medical care. Chapter 4 focuses on explanations for small-area variation and the need to change the behavior of physicians with regard to the use of specific procedures. Dr. Wennberg hypothesizes that there is an inverse relation between the extent of variation in the use of a particular procedure and the degree of consensus among physicians; that is, low-variation procedures are associated with a high consensus among physicians, and high-variation procedures are associated with a low consensus among physicians. For those cases where scientific consensus on the safety and efficacy of a particular treatment is lacking, outcomes should be studied carefully. Patterns of physician practice may be altered by the opinions of peers. However, the absence of definitive information regarding outcomes hinders uniform decision making. Improved documentation of these factors is needed if physicians and patients are to understand the benefits and risks of treatment.

There are those, however, who feel that Dr. Wennberg's explanation of the variation in utilization does little to identify the "causes" of the phenomenon. Among the critics is Dr. Francis Moore, who has written that small-area variation methods are merely a record of the net supply of a procedure to the crude total population of an area. This, he believes, is not an indicator of "practice styles," but rather the net vector of a host of variables.

Chapter 5 offers a critique of analyses of the variation among small areas. Dr. Moore argues that in evaluating clinical care, a statistical base is essential for analysis and interpretation. He focuses on the demand for treatment, the number of treatment options available, and the distribution or frequency of the complaints that bring patients to a physician. His points, supported by specific examples, form the basis of his alternative to the classic theory on small-area variation: treatment options and practice profiles. Dr. Moore believes that patients' complaints mandate a choice among alternative treatments; in his opinion, to assign all treatment variability to "practice style" is not justified. His methodology depends on the selection of a cohort, the evaluation of the use of several treatment options in that cohort, and the expression of ratios that indicate the practice pattern. Comparison of alternative procedures either within a hospital or among several hospitals could be made.

THE CHANGING ENVIRONMENT OF HEALTH CARE

The era of the solo, fee-for-service medical practitioner is slowly dying as the progressively competitive environment of health care reshapes how care is delivered. Consumers are increasingly aware of alternative medical systems and are seeking to "gain control" of their health, to be less passive in their dealings with the medical establishment. The ramifications for surgeons are substantial, since surgery is a costly component of medical care and since questions about the performance of unnecessary surgery abound. New constraints on surgeons will most probably affect the way in which care is delivered and reimbursed.

Understanding the discretionary component in hospital admissions is critical for dealing with the increased demand for service that is likely to accompany the aging of the population. There are large variations in physicians' recommendations for hospitalization that are substantially independent of patients' needs. If appropriate measurements of these variations could be made and the variations then brought into line, the demand for hospital beds could be managed better.

Despite the existence of marked differences in physicians' behaviors, few direct studies of the influence of hospital patterns or of physicians' styles of practice have been carried out. Chapter 6 elucidates the importance of measuring the discretionary element in patterns of hospitalization. Dr. Leslie and Dr. Noralou Roos discuss the significance of such measurement in helping to control hospital costs. They discuss several ways to categorize hospitals and physicians according to the extent to which patients are hospitalized. Since hospitalization is not always in the patient's best interest, discretionary hospital admissions have implications for the quality of care.

Chapter 7 examines the effect of organizational changes on surgical services. Mr. Ermann's review of the proliferation of ambulatory surgery units and multihospital systems looks at the costs and the quality of care in such settings. He addresses the changes in the organization and reimbursement of health services and shows how they have contributed to major shifts in the delivery of surgical services. In our rush to control costs, we must maintain a system that delivers high-quality care. We need to evaluate more fully the implications of these changes in delivery for the cost and quality of care.

A number of studies have documented an inverse relation between a high volume of patients in a hospital for a specific procedure or diagnosis and the number of subsequent deaths or complications. This negative correlation between volume and poor outcome can be due to two possible factors: increased volume results in better outcomes (learning and improving by doing) and a referral effect (a physician or hospital with a better reputation attracts patients). If a better outcome were dependent solely on a higher volume, one could choose a hospital or physician at random and send all patients in a geographical area with a particular diagnosis there. If the relation between volume and outcome is entirely the result of a certain physician's or hospital's having special skills, then regionalization to improve outcome will require an identification of those skilled providers and the referral of patients to them. A patient is more likely to survive a specific surgical procedure when it is performed in a hospital that provides a greater than average number of similar procedures.

The call for the regionalization of surgical services has recently begun to receive attention. Chapter 8 discusses the complexity this issue and the problems of identifying hospitals for regionalization. Dr. Luft and Ms. Hunt utilize case-abstract data for patients having cardiac catheterization performed. They show how data on postsurgical problems can be used to identify superior or inferior care; however, both the volume of operations performed and the skill of the individual physician are important to consider. They suggest that patients could be given an economic incentive to utilize the providers with better outcomes.

THE EFFECT OF NEW TECHNOLOGY ON SURGICAL CARE

Anne Scitovsky has examined the effects of changing medical technologies on the costs of medical care by comparing the costs of treatment of a number of common illnesses during three different periods (1951–64, 1964–71, and 1971–81). While the two earlier time-series studies showed that the main cost-raising change was a steep rise in the use of relatively low-cost ancillary services (laboratory tests and X-rays), the most recent study reveals that the use of these "little ticket" technologies has barely changed but that several new and expensive technologies are increasingly used, which has served to raise the costs of medical care considerably.

Recent technological advances have facilitated successful outcomes of medical procedures as well as complicated and intensified the work of those who are responsible for those procedures. Computerized tomography, ultrasound technology, cardiac catheterization, arteriography, nuclear magnetic resonance, and the introduction of laser therapy have revolutionized many surgical procedures and made possible the development of other procedures that were deemed too risky or dangerous a few years ago.

While advances in medicine and surgery have been facilitated by new technologies, the issue of financial coverage (reimbursement) for new treatments has become more complicated. Third-party payers have the authority to determine whether to pay for procedures involving new medical technology. In the light of the spiraling costs of health care, both private payers and the government are giving new medical technologies increased scrutiny before approving coverage. Decisions regarding coverage for procedures involving new technology depend on whether the treatment is safe and effective. Studies to assess the technology are helpful in making such determinations. The modern concept of technology assessment encompasses an evaluation of the consequences of medical technology, that is, of drugs, devices, equipment, procedures, and support systems used in the care of patients. Technology assessment is meant to be comprehensive, looking at technical performance, clinical efficacy, safety, cost and efficiency, acceptability, and ethics.

Chapter 9 delineates selected federal examinations of medical technologies that include surgery. Dr. Sisk and Ms. Ruby, researchers with the Office of Technology Assessment of the U.S. Congress, elucidate the problems and limitations in the federal process. From political, ethical, and economic perspectives, there is a need for assessment. The inadequacy of the review of surgical techniques is particularly striking.

WHAT LIES AHEAD?

More than $450 billion per year is spent on health care in the United States today; it is estimated that by the year 2000 the costs will escalate to $1 trillion, a sum that is almost incomprehensible. The faulty payment systems that have been driving up costs are being rectified, but other forces continue to generate higher expenditures: changing characteristics of the population, accelerating development and diffusion of new medical technologies, and a heightened pubic expectation for high quality care, contribute to inflation of the costs of medical care.

Profound changes will continue to transform the financing and delivery of health care through the twentieth century. In all likelihood, employers will heighten their demands for high-quality care while managing its utilization and costs. Employers and insurers will monitor the overuse of services, care will be shifted to less costly settings, and sophisticated data bases on the patterns and costs of medical practice will enable purchasers to direct patients to "efficient" providers. As increasing numbers of lay people, both groups and individuals, acquire an interest in the organization of the health care system, the physician's autonomy is eroding. Managed care and the review of utilization are examples of challenges to the traditional authority of the physician.

Chapter 10 tries to summarize the problems confronting surgeons. Research on the utilization of surgical care has raised a number of important questions, the answers to which are not entirely clear. Dr. Roos focuses on policy questions and research needs in the context of current and developing issues.

CONCLUSION

The issues raised in this volume are not easily resolved. A problem in drawing policy conclusions is that, since researchers may approach a question from different perspectives, those studies that have been conducted make conflicting recommendations. Additionally, whereas the data on costs and utilization are easily analyzed and understood, the data on quality and outcomes are often more difficult to assess. Indeed, care delivered must be closely monitored to insure that in the rush to contain costs, we maintain a system delivering high quality care.

1 Surgical Care in Developed Nations

Eugene Vayda, M.D., and Janet M. Barnsley, M.E.S.

Substantial cross-national variation in surgical rates has been reported regularly and consistently since the 1960s. Some studies have identified statistical correlations between higher rates and fee-for-service payment, greater numbers of hospital beds, surgical staff, resources devoted to medical care, and consumer preferences. "Unnecessary surgery" has been suggested as one possible cause of the differences in rates (1).

This chapter compares the surgical rates of developed nations. Both national and regional data within countries have been examined and correlations with possible causative factors are described. Other chapters will review regional variations in the United States and variations within small areas in the United States and elsewhere.

A number of studies have classified operations into two general categories: primarily discretionary and primarily nondiscretionary. The former category includes tonsil surgery, varicose vein stripping, cataract surgery, and hysterectomy. (Less than 10 percent of hysterectomies in Canada are done for malignant disease, for example.) Nondiscretionary procedures are those in which a patient's or physician's choice is usually not a factor, for example, pneumonectomy, appendectomy. This classification was developed to test the hypothesis that there would be less variation in rates in the primarily nondiscretionary category. However, this has not always proven to be the case. Many procedures are done in both discretionary and nondiscretionary circumstances (e.g., herniorrhaphy: elective versus strangulation or incarceration; cholecystectomy: asymptomatic gallstones versus jaundice or carcinoma). There is also considerable controversy regarding the dis-

---

The preparation of this chapter was supported in part by a grant from Physicians Services Incorporated Foundation, Toronto, Ontario, Canada.

cretionary/nondiscretionary status of operations such as coronary artery bypass, thyroidectomy for hyperthyroidism, and surgery for herniated intervertebral disc disease.

One major problem with the interpretation of cross-national studies is that data are frequently collected and reported differently in the countries examined. Most of the cross-national studies have attempted to standardize the data from the countries they compare. Instances where standardization is difficult are usually identified but frequently not dealt with adequately: day surgery, private surgery in the United Kingdom, surgery in the armed forces, changing classification or nomenclature from one International Classification of Disease Adapted (ICDA) edition to the next. Standardization is even more of a problem when data from different studies are compared. However, the magnitude of the variation between countries is so great and so consistent that the presence of true cross-national differences cannot be seriously questioned, although the causes are still not fully understood.

Variables that have been suggested as causes of the differences are even harder to standardize. Total numbers of hospital beds are difficult to measure because each country uses a separate classification. As well, countries count numbers of surgeons differently. When measured at all, consumer preferences are not determined in the same ways in different studies. Correlations with differing methods of organizing and paying for surgical care are frequently confounded by other variables (2).

Rates are usually calculated using population denominators rather than the incidence or prevalence of the conditions for which the surgery is done. Almost none of the studies takes the concept of "population at risk for organ loss" into consideration (3). Once an organ has been removed, a patient is no longer at risk for the removal of that organ although he or she is still counted in the population denominator.

THE EARLY STUDIES

Several early studies reported crude rates, but many of the operations and their associated conditions are age and sex related. This problem has been addressed by calculating age and sex-specific or standardized operative rates.

In 1965 Logan and Eimerl reported a comparison of Saskatchewan, Canada; New England, United States; Liverpool, England; and Sodertalje, Sweden (4). Crude rates were reported for six common procedures. Liverpool ranked lowest for them all. Saskatchewan was highest for tonsil surgery; New England and Saskatchewan were highest for hysterectomy and hemorrhoidectomy; and Sweden had the highest rates for cholecystectomy, varicose vein surgery, and prostatectomy. There was a sixfold variation for cholecystectomy, a fourfold variation in tonsil surgery rates, and a threefold variation for varicose vein surgery and hemorrhoidectomy.

Two years later Pearson and others (5) reported a comparison that included Liverpool, England; New England, United States; and Uppsala, Sweden (5). They found that sex- and age-specific rates in New England for common primarily nondiscretionary operations such as tonsil surgery, hysterectomy, and inguinal herniorrhaphy were twice those in Uppsala and Liverpool.

Although cities and regions do not necessarily reflect national trends, subsequent international comparisons have confirmed the findings reported by Pearson and colleagues and by Logan and Eimerl. Bunker compared England and Wales in 1966 with the United States in 1965 (6). The crude overall U.S. operative rate was twice that in England and Wales. There were twofold to threefold differences for Pearson's three primarily discretionary operations and similar differences for several others (the rate of cholecystectomy in the United States was 3 times that in England and Wales; and hemorrhoidectomies were performed 4 times more often in the United States).

A subsequent one-year study of Canada (1968) and England and Wales (1967) by Vayda found that the overall Canadian rate was 1.7 times that of England and Wales (7). Age-standardized sex-specific rates for common primarily nondiscretionary operations were 2 or more times greater in Canada than in England and Wales. Cholecystectomy in women was almost 7 times greater in Canada. The higher Canadian gallbladder surgery incidence was confirmed by Plant and others (8). His group compared gallbladder surgery rates in three similar towns in Canada, France, and England. The cholecystectomy rate in one Canadian town in 1971 was 6 times higher than the rates in the two European towns (9 times higher for patients under age thirty-five). Cholecystectomy rates in all three towns doubled between 1961 and 1971.

The Vayda Study also reported that the Canadian mortality rate for gallbladder disease in women forty-five and older was 1.8 times higher than that in England and Wales (7). It raised the question of whether the higher mortality was due to greater gallbladder disease mortality or to surgically related mortality, and concluded that at least part of the variation was due to the surgery. Mortality for uterine and cervical cancer was identical in the two countries, although the Canadian hysterectomy rate was 2.2 times the England and Wales rate. Mortality from breast cancer was 10 percent lower in Canada in the face of a Canadian radical mastectomy rate, which was 3.2 times the England and Wales rate.

MORE RECENT STUDIES

The four early studies were based on single-year analyses, and although the differences were consistent, they could have been due to chance variation. To deal with this possibility, Vayda, Mindell, and Rutkow carried out a ten-year (1966–76) analysis of surgical rates in Canada, the United States, and England and Wales (9). Age- and sex-adjusted rates (with normal obstetrics and diagnostic procedures removed) were examined in three ways: overall rates, rates for specific ICDA-8 surgical chapters, and rates for specific operations. Overall rates averaged about 4,000 per 100,000 people in England and Wales, about 6,200 in Canada, and in the United States just over 7,000 in 1966 and almost 9,000 in 1976. The rankings of the three countries were the same for all the ICDA-8 surgical chapters (England and Wales lowest, Canada intermediate, and United States highest). England and Wales were lowest for all the individual operations studied, and the United States was highest for all except tonsil and gallbladder surgery.

The countrywide and cross-national trends for categories of operations and for individual operations over the seven-year period from 1970 to 1976 were of particular interest. Neurosurgery and orthopedic surgery increased in all three countries (but increased the least in England and Wales). Eye surgery increased in Canada and the United States, largely as a result of increases in lens extraction. In England and Wales both eye surgery and lens extraction remained unchanged. Otolaryngologic surgery remained the same in the United States but decreased 20 percent in Canada and England and Wales, with a substantial decrease in tonsil surgery in all three countries: 23 percent in the United States, 35 percent in England and Wales, and 41 percent in Canada.

Abdominal surgery changed only slightly, with small reductions in England and Wales (2 percent) and Canada (9 percent) and a small increase (11 percent) in the United States. Inguinal herniorrhaphy decreased in all three countries, yet decreased the most (12 percent) in England and Wales, which started the decade 40 percent lower than Canada and the United States. Canada ranked highest for cholecystectomy (2 times the United States rate and 5.6 times that in England and Wales), and its rate fell 20 percent from 1970 to 1976, while both England and Wales and the United States registered increases of about 12 percent.

Gynecologic surgery showed small changes in England and Wales (12 percent decrease) and Canada (7 percent increase) and a substantial increase in the United States (33 percent). The increase in the United States was due largely to an 18 percent increase in hysterectomy (both Canada and England and Wales had small decreases) and a 126 percent increase in cesarean section. Cesarean section increased 83 percent in Canada and 53 percent in England and Wales. By 1976 the rate of cesarean section (per 100 live births) was 12.0 in the US, 10.6 in Canada, 6.6 in England and Wales.

Cesarean section is of particular interest because the reported rates are based on the incidence of the condition being treated (live births) and are not influenced by the problem of "population at risk for organ loss." However, cross-national rankings for cesarean section were the same as those for the other procedures studied. Rates in England and Wales were the lowest, and increased the least. The United States had the highest rates, and the greatest increase, and the Canadian rate and increase were intermediate.

A cross-national comparison of 1975 mortality rates for conditions associated with the operations studied was also done (table 1.1). The United States and England and Wales had similar death rates for gallbladder diseases despite the fact that their cholecystectomy rates varied by almost 300 percent. Canada's death rate for gallbladder diseases and its cholecystectomy rates were both highest. England and Wales had the lowest prostatectomy rates and the lowest mortality for prostatic carcinoma and hyperplasia. On the other hand, in England and Wales mortality for malignant disease of the breast was highest and those countries had the lowest breast surgery rates. The hysterectomy rates were twice as high in Canada and the United States as in England and Wales. However, the three countries had comparable mortality rates for malignant disease of the female genital tract in women age sixty-five and older, but in England and Wales mortality for women between ages forty-five and sixty-four was approximately 25 percent higher than in Canada or the United States.

On a per capita basis, England and Wales had the lowest number of beds and the lowest operative rates. In 1974 and 1976, Canada had 30 percent more hospital beds than the United States, but overall operative rates were 40 percent higher in the United States than in Canada.

Surgeon numbers, like overall operative rates, were lowest in England and Wales, intermediate in Canada, and highest in the United States during the entire study period. Overall surgical rates in Canada and England and Wales remained constant despite small per capita increases in numbers of surgeons. In the United States, both the operative rates and numbers of surgeons increased; although between 1974 and 1976, the surgeon-to-population ratio increased more rapidly than the surgical rate.

Comparable expenditure data as percentages of gross national product (GNP) spent on health care are available for the United States,

TABLE 1.1. Age- and Sex-Specific Mortality for Selected Conditions: Canada, England and Wales, and the United States, 1975

			Rates per 100,000 People		
Cause of Death	ICDA-8 Codes	Sex/Age Group/Yr	Canada	England and Wales	U.S.A.
Malignant neoplasm of the breast	174	F-45/64	68	80	64
		F-65	124	141	114
Hernia with/without obstruct. intest.	550	M-45–64	2	3	2
	553	M-65	22	26	19
Obstruct. no hernia	560				
Cholelithiasis	574	F-45–64	1	1	1
Cholecystitis, without calculus	575	F-65	17	12	11
Hyperplasia of prostate	600	M-45–64	10	10	12
Cancer of prostate	185	M-65	216	179	199
Colon cancer	153	M-45–64	25	24	28
Diverticula	562	M-65	149	124	144
Enteritis, ulcerative colitis	563				
Cancer of cervix; uterus, ovaries, fallopian tubes, broad ligament	180–83	F-45–64	37	51	40
		F-65	80	87	83
Cancer of urinary organs	189	M-45–64	8	7	9
		M-65	27	22	25

Source: Reference 9. Reprinted with permission of publisher.

Canada, and the United Kingdom (England, Wales, Scotland, and Northern Ireland) (10). During the decade from 1966 to 1976, the United Kingdom spent between 4.3 and 5.8 percent of its GNP on health care, Canada 6.1 to 7.2 percent, and the United States 5.8 to 8.6 percent. From 1970 onward, the GNP expenditure rankings mirrored the rankings for overall surgical rates in the three countries. In the 1970s, the United Kingdom increased its percentage of GNP spent on health care although surgical rates in England and Wales remained constant; in Canada, both the overall rates and GNP percentages were unchanged; and in the United States, both increased substantially.

McPherson, Strong, and Epstein compared eight common operations in England and Wales, Canada, and the United States in 1975 (11). Six had been included in the ten-year comparison described above (hysterectomy, cholecystectomy, prostatectomy, tonsil surgery, herniorrhaphy, lens extraction). Because the McPherson study used a different reference standard, its age- and sex-standardized rates were

TABLE 1.2. Possible Sources of Variations in Rates of Surgery based on Geographic Areas

1. Age and sex composition
2. Age-specific disease incidence
3. Random variation with time and place
4. Availability
   A. Manpower
   B. Hospital bed provision
   C. Funding
   D. Waiting lists
   E. Methods of payment
5. Clinical judgment
6. Variations in patient demand or expectation
7. Rates of organ removal in previous years
8. Prevailing custom
9. Systematic omissions of operations, e.g., Private surgery day cases
10. Differences in coding procedures
11. Inaccuracies in information sources

Source: Reference 11. Reprinted with permission of publisher.

somewhat different from those reported in the ten-year study, but differences of the same magnitude for the six common operations are noted in both studies. McPherson also examined regional variations in the three countries and found considerable regional variation. However, if we exclude the smallest Canadian province (Prince Edward Island, population approximately 120,000), McPherson's highest regional rate in England and Wales is still lower than the lowest regional rate in Canada or the United States for five of the six operations common to both studies (with the exception of lens extraction).

McPherson and colleagues also systematically reviewed the various possible sources of variation in rates of surgery in different geographic areas (table 1.2) and attempted to explain variation in their reported rates using these variables. Although they were able to explain between 54 and 86 percent of the regional variation in surgical rates for their eight operations, only a few explanatory variables common to several procedures emerged, for example, waiting time (variously classified) and manpower (number of surgeons). Except for resources, the explanatory variables listed in table 1.2 have not been consistently measured in the reported studies or consistently associated with variation in rates in cross-national studies.

In a companion study, McPherson and others reported 1975 age- and sex-standardized rates for seven of the previously studied eight operations (all except lens extraction) in one region of England and Wales, three New England states, and southern Norway (12). Southern Norway's operative rates occupied a variable but generally low position when compared to England and Wales and the United States (lowest for cholecystectomy, tonsillectomy, hysterectomy, and intermediate for the remaining four operations).

A more recent review of cesarean section rates and perinatal mortality in eleven countries in Europe and North America in 1979–80 showed fourfold variation between the highest and lowest countries (13). Czechoslovakia had the lowest cesarean rate (4.0) and the highest perinatal mortality rate (PMR) (18.4). Cesarean section rates in England and Wales (8.8) and Scotland (10.7) were intermediate and were accompanied by PMRs above the average for the eleven countries (15.7 and 14.2, respectively). On the other hand, lower or intermediate cesarean rates were accompanied by low PMRs in the Netherlands (12.0), Denmark (9.8), Norway (11.9), and Sweden (9.1). Canada's cesarean rate (15.2 in 1980) was among the highest, but its perinatal mortality rate (10.8) was comparable to the PMRs in the Netherlands, Denmark, Norway, and Sweden, four countries with lower cesarean rates.

NEXT STEPS

Rates in the developed countries reported have been sustained and consistent, primarily for nondiscretionary operations. The differences are tolerated without obvious or consistent unfavorable outcomes or consumer dissatisfaction. Treatment styles and therapeutic indications have changed (e.g., reductions in tonsil surgery and increases in cesarean sections). England and Wales and other European countries had lower rates generally than Canada or the United States, and except for gallbladder and tonsil surgery, Canada's rates are lower than those in the United States. Although national rates are still monitored, emphasis today is shifting toward regional and small-area comparisons (studies of differing surgical treatment styles and practices at the community level) (14), toward identifying a research agenda that will determine efficacy of surgical treatments, and as a result of such efficacy studies, toward modifying physician behavior. Regional and small-area comparisons afford a better opportunity than cross-national studies to identify variables that may contribute causally to differing rates. Roos and Roos have shown that a complete and reliable regionwide data set, which includes morbidity, utilization, number of surgeons, and resource information, can demonstrate consistent statistical associations between these variables and rates for specific operations (15,16). Generally, more resources have been associated with higher surgical rates.

Community-based studies can more readily examine practice styles, which are more difficult to measure in large-scale studies and in those using existing data sets. While higher operative rates may, to some degree, mean unnecessary surgery, optimal levels of surgery for particular diagnoses are still not well established. Community-based studies must be coupled with well-designed studies of natural history and of efficacy of individual operations for specific diseases or syndromes. Gracie and Ranshoff's recent report is one example, a study that questions cholecystectomy for asymptomatic gallstones. There are other examples where established surgical and medical procedures, when subjected to scrutiny, have been discarded (18,19). On the other hand, the finding that cesarean section rates in the Canadian province of Ontario ranged between 3.8 and 16.6 per 100 live births in 1977 (20) coupled with the comparable fourfold variation reported in cesarean rates in the eleven-country study (13) probably indicates that excessive and suboptimal levels of surgery coexist in different countries or a single province.

There are many instances where existing evidence supporting or rejecting particular surgical or nonsurgical treatments has not been incorporated into clinical practice. The practice of mandatory repeat cesarean section is not supported by the existing evidence although it is almost universally followed (95 percent in Ontario). A recent Canadian Consensus Conference found no evidence to support the practice of "once a section always a section" (21). The conference recommendations for more trials of labor in women with a single previous low transverse section could, with proper dissemination, result in a change in physician behavior and a decrease (in some locations) in cesarean rates.

POLICY OPTIONS

Cross-national surgical studies have played a major part in initiating dialogue regarding necessary and unnecessary surgery and in clarifying the factors involved in physician and patient choices. Cross-national differences continue to be a subject for discussion and concern (22). While continued monitoring to detect, measure, and publicize trends is essential, controversy over necessary and unnecessary surgery can only be resolved with the dissemination of results from appropriately designed efficacy studies and the monitoring of clinical practice. Cross-national studies opened the doors and made us aware of problems that now require more detailed examination and resolution.

Even after inappropriate surgical use is identified, the mechanisms that modify provider behavior differ from country to country, although provider and consumer education can be employed regardless of how services are organized or paid for. In Canada, with national health insurance and fee-for-service payment, the government–medical society negotiated fee schedules could be used to increase or decrease specific types of utilization. It has been suggested that the fee for elective cesarean in cases of previous low transverse section should be reduced and the fee for management by trial of labor increased. In the United States, individual third-party payers could employ similar approaches or put in place incentives based on diagnosis-related groups (DRGs). In England, with universal health insurance and salaried surgeons, national and regional standards and hospital-based peer review and monitoring may be appropriate strategies. Consensus conferences based on careful analysis of existing evidence are already used as preliminary steps to modify provider behavior in the United States (23), Canada (21), and the United Kingdom (24).

REFERENCES

1. Rutkow, I.M. Unnecessary surgery: What is it? *Surg Clin N Amer* 62:613–25 (1982).
2. Crymble, C., and Vayda, E. Surgical rates in the Canadian forces and the general Canadian population. *Clin Invest Med* 4:37–40 (1981).
3. Gittelsohn, A.M., and Wennberg, J.E. On the risk of organ loss. *J Chron Dis* 29:527–35 (1976).
4. Logan, R.F.L., and Eimerl, T.S. Case loads in hospitals and general practice in several countries. *In:* Acheson, R.M., ed., *Comparability in International Epidemiology.* New York: Milbank Memorial Fund 302-10 (1964).
5. Pearson, R.J.C., Smedbey, B., Berfenstam, R., et al. Hospital caseloads in Liverpool, New England, and Uppsala: An international comparison. *Lancet* 2:559–66 (1968).
6. Bunker, J.P. Surgical manpower: A comparison of operation and surgeons in the United States and England and Wales. *N Eng J Med* 282:135–44 (1970).
7. Vayda, E. A comparison of surgical rates in Canada and in England and Wales. *N Eng J Med* 289:1224–29 (1973).
8. Plant, J.C.D., Percy, I., Bates, T., et al. Incidence of gallbladder disease in Canada, England, and France. *Lancet* 2:249–51 (1973).
9. Vayda, E., Mindell, W.R., and Rutkow, I.M. A decade of surgery in Canada, England and Wales, and the United States. *Arch Surg* 117:846–53 (1982).
10. Simanis, J.G., and Coleman, J.R. Health care expenditures in nine industrialized countries, 1960–1976. *Soc Sec Bull* 43:3–8 (1980).
11. McPherson, K., Strong, P.M., Epstein, A., et al. Regional variations in the use of common surgical procedures within and between England and Wales, Canada, and the United States of America. *Soc Sci and Med* 273–88 (1981).
12. McPherson, K., Wennberg, J.E., Hovind, O.B., et al. Small-area variations

in the use of common surgical procedures: An international comparison of New England, England, and Norway. *N Eng J Med* 307:1310–14 (1982).
13. Loma, J., and Enkin, M. Variations in operative delivery rates. *In:* Enkin, M., Chalmers, I., Keirse, M., eds., *Effective Care in Pregnancy and Childbirth.* London: Oxford University Press (1987).
14. Wennberg, J.E., and Gittelsohn, A.M. Small-area variations in health care delivery. *Science* 182:1102–8 (1973).
15. Roos, N.P., and Roos, L.L. High and low surgical rates: Risk factors for area residents. *Am J Pub Hlth* 71:591–600 (1981).
16. Roos, L.L. Supply, workload, and utilization: A population-based analysis of surgery in rural Manitoba. *Am J Pub Hlth* 73:414–21 (1983).
17. Gracie, W.A., and Ranshoff, D.F. The natural history of silent gallstones: The innocent gallstone is not a myth. *N Eng J Med* 798–800 (1982).
18. Barsamian, E.M. The rise and fall of internal mammary artery litigation in the treatment of angina pectoris and the lessons learned. *In:* Bunker, J.P., Barnes, B.A., Mosteller, F., eds., *Costs, Risks, and Benefits of Surgery.* New York: Oxford University Press (1977).
19. Lin Miao, L. Gastric freezing: An example of the evaluation of medical therapy by randomized clinical trials. *In:* Bunker, J.P., Barnes, B.A., Mosteller, F., eds., *Costs, Risks, and Benefits of Surgery.* New York: Oxford University Press (1977).
20. Vayda, E., Barnsley, J.M., Mindell, W.R., et al. Five-year study of surgical rates in Ontario's counties. *Can Med Assoc J* 131:111–15 (1984).
21. Hannah, W.J. Indications for cesarean section: Final statement of the panel of the National Consensus on Aspects of Cesarean Birth. *Can Med Assoc J* 134:1348–52 (1986).
22. Lohr, K., Lohr, W.R., and Brook, R.H. Understanding variations in the use of services: Are there clinical explanations? *Health Policy* 3:139–47 (1984).
23. Jacoby, I. The consensus development program of the National Institutes of Health: Current practices and historical perspectives. *Int J Tech Assess Health Care* 2:420–32 (1985).
24. Stocking, B. First consensus development conference in the United Kingdom: On coronary artery bypass grafting. 1: Views of audience, panel, and speakers. *Br Med J (Clin Res)* 291:713–16 (1985).

2 Surgical Operations and Manpower Considerations

Ira M. Rutkow, M.D., Dr.P.H.

The 1970s and 1980s have marked a period of active social change. This has been especially true for all branches of surgery, as witnessed, for example by the growing debate over "unnecessary surgery" (1–2). Claims of large increases in the number of surgical operations have elicited concern (3). Quite clearly, surgery has increased, but to what extent, and is the increase continuing? The issue of the number of surgeons in the United States has also been the focus of much debate and discussion (4–5). Many questions remain unanswered: What changes can we expect to see, what adjustments will be required as a result of the unprecedented number of surgeons being trained in the United States? What constitutes an appropriate caseload for practicing surgeons?

This chapter addresses these issues by analyzing the number of surgical operations and surgeon population statistics for the five-year periods 1970–74 and 1979–83; by listing the ten most frequently performed operations for each specialty in 1983; by reviewing previous attempts to quantify and determine appropriate patient-physician ratios; and by providing specific recommendations for setting future staffing needs.

In an attempt to address unanswered questions, I utilized surgical rate data compiled by the National Center for Health Statistics. Findings from the period 1979–83 were compared with data for the years 1970–74 (6–10). Since 1965, the National Center for Health Statistics has compiled data on the number of surgical operations performed annually (11). The sample data were expanded to produce estimates of the absolute number of operations performed nationally by age and sex in a given year, although results are subject to both nonsampling and sampling errors. The approximate relative standard errors of estimated numbers of procedures employed herein are as follows: 10,000 operations, 18 percent; 100,000 operations, 11 percent; 1,000,000 operations, 7 percent; and 10,000,000 operations, 5 percent (12).

In analyzing the total number of surgical operations, the growing concept of outpatient or ambulatory surgery must be considered (13). There are three basic outpatient unit models: hospital-based, nondedicated units; hospital-based, defined units; and the freestanding unit. Hospital Discharge Survey data include most operations performed in hospital-based outpatient units. For this chapter, "minor" outpatient operations that may be performed in a hospital's operating room are excluded, as are surgical operations performed in freestanding units. In 1983, there were approximately 370 freestanding surgical units in which 350,000 ambulatory operations were performed. This figure represents only 2 percent of all surgical operations performed (14).

In my analysis, the ten most frequently performed surgical procedures for each specialty were selected for the years 1979, 1981, and 1983. The assignment of an operation or group of operations to a particular surgical specialty was based on generally accepted ICDA-9-CM groupings. Plastic surgery and colon and rectal surgery could not be individually studied since they have no separate ICDA-9-CM codes. Additionally, even though an operation is listed within a particular specialty, it does not necessarily mean that all or nearly all of those operations were performed by members of that subspecialty. For example, excision of an intervertebral disc is assigned to orthopedic surgery even though neurosurgeons may often perform surgery for this condition.

To analyze surgical "manpower," the number of surgical operations should be linked with the number of physicians who perform those operations. To accomplish this, I consulted the American Medical Association's *Physician Distribution and Medical Licensure* (PDML) reference guide. The reference guide does not provide information on how many surgeons are actually performing surgery, how many have retired, how many are on fellowships, or how many are in administrative roles.

STATISTICAL EVIDENCE

In 1970, a total of 12,550,000 surgical operations were performed in the United States. By 1974, the figure had increased to 15,663,000, more than 25 percent. During this same period, there was an 8 percent increase in the total number of surgeons in the country. In 1979, 17,065,000 surgical operations were performed; in 1983, 18,550,000 operations were performed, an increase of more than 9 percent. During this five-year period, there was a 19 percent increase in the total number of surgeons.

In 1970, the number of surgical cases per surgeon was 187. This peaked in 1974 at 217. By 1979, it had decreased to 176, and five years later the rate had dropped to 161. Although there was spectacular growth in numbers of operations during the early and mid 1970s, it is apparent that the numbers of operations and cases per surgeon have decreased enormously over the last five to ten years. On average, a surgeon today performs three operations per week.

General Surgery

In 1970, a total of 3,755,000 general surgical operations were completed. By 1974, this had increased to 4,370,000, a change of 16 percent. During this five-year period, there was a 5 percent increase in the total number of physicians who labeled themselves general surgeons. In 1979, 4,729,000 general surgical operations were performed with an increase to 5,041,000 in 1983. This represents a 7 percent change. During this five-year period, there was a 13 percent increase in the number of physicians who labeled themselves general surgeons. (Table 2.1 lists the ten most frequently performed procedures.)

In 1970, the number of surgical cases per general surgeon was 166. This peaked in 1974 at 184. By 1979, the rate had decreased to 148 cases per surgeon, and five years later it was down to 139.

Obstetrics-Gynecology

In 1970, 2,841,000 obstetric-gynecologic operations were performed. By 1974, this had increased to 3,987,000, a rise of 40 percent. During this five-year period, there was a 7 percent increase in the total number of physicians who labeled themselves obstetrician-gynecologists.

In 1979, 4,339,000 obstetric-gynecologic operations were performed, with a 1 percent decrease to 4,304,000 in 1983. During this five-year period, there was a 22 percent increase in the number of

TABLE 2.1. The Ten Most Frequent General Surgical Operations

Procedure	1983 Total	1979 Total
1. Inguinal hernia	585,000	579,000
2. Cholecystectomy	487,000	445,000
3. Lysis of peritoneal adhesions	298,000	259,000
4. Appendectomy	282,000	311,000
5. Biopsy or local excision of breast lesion	233,000	323,000
6. Debridement of wound, burn, or infection	219,000	164,000
7. Partial excision of large intestine	169,000	133,000
8. Hemorrhoidectomy	129,000	164,000
9. Free skin graft	120,000	126,000
10. Mastectomy	116,000	112,000

TABLE 2.2. The Ten Most Frequent Obstetric-Gynecologic Operations

Procedure	1983 Total	1979 Total
1. Cesarean section	809,000	601,000
2. Hysterectomy	673,000	638,000
3. Diagnostic dilation and curettage	632,000	935,000
4. Open destruction or occlusion of fallopian tubes	568,000	547,000
5. Salpingo-oophorectomy	457,000	400,000
6. Diagnostic laparoscopy	262,000	203,000
7. Repair of cystocele and rectocele	150,000	175,000
8. Local excision of ovarian lesion	107,000	92,000
9. Endoscopic destruction or occlusion of fallopian tubes	105,000	196,000
10. Conization of cervix	71,000	88,000

physicians who labeled themselves obstetrician-gynecologists. (Table 2.2 lists the ten most frequently performed procedures.)

In 1970, the number of surgical cases per obstetrician-gynecologist was 174. This peaked in 1974 at 227. By 1979, it had decreased to 181, and five years later the rate was 147.

Orthopedic Surgery

In 1970, a total of 2,005,000 orthopedic operations were completed. By 1974, this had increased to 2,576,000, for a change of 28 percent. During this five-year period, there was a 15 percent increase in the total number of physicians who labeled themselves orthopedic surgeons.

In 1979, 2,858,000 orthopedic operations were performed with an increase to 3,549,000 by 1983. This represents a 24 percent change. During this five-year period, there was a 28 percent increase in numbers of physicians who label themselves orthopedic surgeons. (Table 2.3 lists the ten most frequently performed procedures.)

In 1970, the number of surgical cases per orthopedic surgeon was 258. This peaked in 1974, when it was 288. By 1979, it had decreased to 226 and five years later was down to 219.

TABLE 2.3. The Ten Most Frequent Orthopedic Operations

Procedure	1983 Total	1979 Total
1. Open reduction with internal fixation	331,000	274,000
2. Arthroscopy	260,000	130,000
3. Excision of intervertebral disc	188,000	132,000
4. Closed reduction without internal fixation	183,000	238,000
5. Excision of bunion	182,000	112,000
6. Placement or removal of internal-fixation device without fracture reduction	173,000	160,000
7. Arthroplasty of knee and ankle	161,000	123,000
8. Total hip and/or arthroplasty of hip	159,000	130,000
9. Excision of semilunar cartilage of knee	147,000	155,000
10. Local excision of lesion or tissue of bone	136,000	95,000

Otorhinolaryngology

In 1970, a total of 1,687,000 ear-nose-throat (ENT) operations were completed. By 1974, this had increased to 1,838,000, a change of 9 percent. During this five-year period, there was a 5 percent increase in the number of physicians who labeled themselves ENT surgeons.

In 1979, 1,816,000 ENT operations were performed, with a decrease to 1,719,000 in 1983. This represents a decrease of 5 percent. During this five-year period, there was a 15 percent increase in the number of physicians who labeled themselves ENT surgeons. (Table 2.4 lists the ten most frequently performed procedures.)

In 1970, the number of surgical cases per ENT surgeon was 367. This peaked in 1974 at 381. By 1979, the rate had decreased to 297, and five years later it was 244.

Urology

In 1970, a total of 1,221,000 urologic operations were completed. By 1974, this had increased to 1,512,000, a change of 24 percent. During this five-year period, there was a 10 percent increase in the total number of physicians who labeled themselves urologic surgeons.

In 1979, 1,576,000 urologic operations were performed, with an increase to 1,680,000 in 1983. This represents a change of 6 percent. During this five-year period, there was an 18 percent increase in the number of physicians who labeled themselves urologic surgeons. (Table 2.5 lists the ten most frequently performed procedures.)

In 1970, the number of surgical cases per urologic surgeon was 246. This peaked in 1974 at 277. By 1979, it had decreased to 218 and five years later was 197.

Ophthalmology

In 1970, a total of 566,000 ophthalmologic operations were completed. By 1974, this had increased 26 percent to 715,000. During this five-year period, there was an 8 percent increase in the total number of physicians who labeled themselves ophthalmologic surgeons.

In 1979, 815,000 ophthalmologic operations were performed, with an increase to 1,073,000 in 1983. This represents a 32 percent change. During this five-year period, there was a 20 percent increase in the number of physicians who labeled themselves ophthalmologic surgeons. (Table 2.6 lists the ten most frequently performed proceudres.)

In 1970, the number of surgical cases per ophthalmologic surgeons was 66. This peaked in 1974, when it was 77. By 1979, the rate had decreased to 68, but five years later it had risen to 75.

TABLE 2.4. The Ten Most Frequent ENT Operations

Procedure	1983 Total	1979 Total
1. Tonsillectomy	478,000	584,000
2. Repair and plastic operation on the nose	263,000	242,000
3. Myringotomy	187,000	225,000
4. Turbinectomy	90,000	58,000
5. Excision and plastic repair of mouth/lip	57,000	56,000
6. Excision of lesion of nose	50,000	53,000
7. Submucous resection of nasal septum	49,000	59,000
8. Temporary tracheostomy	49,000	42,000
9. Reduction of nasal fracture	37,000	44,000
10. Myringoplasty	37,000	52,000

TABLE 2.5. The Ten Most Frequent Urologic Operations

Procedure	1983 Total	1979 Total
1. Prostatectomy	357,000	293,000
2. Transurethral excision of bladder tissue	135,000	120,000
3. Circumcision (excludes newborn)	91,000	102,000
4. Excision of hydrocele of tunica vaginalis	54,000	49,000
5. Ureterotomy	53,000	41,000
6. Orchiectomy	52,000	42,000
7. Transurethral removal of obstruction from ureter and renal pelvis	52,000	46,000
8. Retropubic urethral suspension	47,000	45,000
9. Release of urethral stricture	45,000	29,000
10. Partial and/or complete nephrectomy	38,000	32,000

TABLE 2.6. The Ten Most Frequent Ophthalmologic Operations

Procedure	1983 Total	1979 Total
1. Extraction of lens	630,000	417,000
2. Repair of retinal tear of detachment	60,000	33,000
3. Operations on extraocular muscles	51,000	66,000
4. Reconstruction of eyelid with flaps, grafts, etc.	40,000	52,000
5. Operations on vitreous	38,000	22,000
6. Excision of lesion of eyelid	27,000	26,000
7. Secondary insertion of intraocular lens	21,000	2,000
8. Corneal trannsplant	20,000	8,000
9. Repair of blepharoptosis and lid retraction	14,000	13,000
10. Scleral fistulization	13,000	14,000

Thoracic and Cardiovascular Surgery

In 1970, a total of 258,000 thoracic and cardiovascular operations were completed. By 1974, this had increased to 349,000, for a change of 35 percent. In 1979, 479,000 thoracic and cardiovascular operations were performed, with an increase to 644,000 in 1983. This represents a 34 percent change. The PDML guide did not report statistics on the number of thoracic and cardiovascular surgeons until the 1980s. Therefore it is not possible to establish case-surgeon ratios. (Table 2.7 lists the ten most frequently performed procedures.)

TABLE 2.7. The Ten Most Frequent Thoracic and Cardiovascular Operations

Procedure	1983 Total	1979 Total
1. Coronary artery bypass	191,000	114,000
2. Insertion, replacement, revision, or removal of pacemaker system	190,000	172,000
3. Incision of mediastinum, mediastinoscopy, or mediastinal biopsy	44,000	33,000
4. Lobectomy of lung	28,000	22,000
5. Removal of coronary artery obstruction	26,000	2,000
6. Excision of tissue of lung	20,000	14,000
7. Replacement of aortic valve	16,000	17,000
8. Replacement of mitral valve	16,000	11,000
9. Implantation or removal of heart assist system	14,000	9,000
10. Repair of atrial and ventricular septa	9,000	7,000

Neurosurgery

In 1970, a total of 217,000 neurosurgical operations were completed. By 1974, this had increased to 316,000, for a change of 46 percent. During this five-year period, there was an 11 percent increase in the number of physicians who labeled themselves neurosurgeons.

In 1979, 453,000 neurosurgical operations were performed, with an increase to 545,000 in 1983. This represents a 20 percent change. During this five-year period, there was a 25 percent increase in the number of physicians who labeled themselves neurosurgeons. (Table 2.8 lists the ten most frequently performed procedures.)

In 1970, the number of surgical cases per neurosurgeon was 105. By 1974, it was 138. In 1979, it peaked at 146. Five years later it had decreased to 141.

TABLE 2.8. The Ten Most Frequent Neurosurgical Operations

Procedure	1983 Total	1979 Total
1. Lysis of adhesions and decompression of peripheral and cranial nerves (includes carpal and tarsal tunnel)	104,000	101,000
2. Exploration and decompression of spinal canal structure	98,000	70,000
3. Incision, division, and excision of peripheral and cranial nerve	69,000	60,000
4. Incision and excision of brain and cerebral meninges	45,000	33,000
5. Craniotomy and craniectomy	36,000	43,000
6. Extracranial ventricular shunt	36,000	21,000
7. Suture and neuroplasty of peripheral and cranial nerve	32,000	31,000
8. Sympathectomy	19,000	22,000
9. Transposition of peripheral and cranial nerves	13,000	7,000
10. Cranioplasty	12,000	13,000

A summary of the preceding data highlights the thirty-five most common operations in the United States for 1983:

1.	Cesarean section	809,000
2.	Hysterectomy	673,000
3.	Diagnostic dilation and curettage of uterus	632,000
4.	Cataract extraction	630,000
5.	Inguinal hernia	585,000
6.	Open destruction of fallopian tubes	568,000
7.	Cholecystectomy	487,000
8.	Tonsillectomy	478,000
9.	Salpingo-oophorectomy	457,000
10.	Prostatectomy	357,000
11.	Open reduction of fracture with internal fixation	331,000
12.	Lysis of peritoneal adhesions	298,000
13.	Appendectomy	282,000
14.	Repair and plastic operations on nose	263,000
15.	Diagnostic laparoscopy	262,000
16.	Arthroscopy	260,000
17.	Biopsy or local excision of breast lesion	233,000
18.	Debridement of wounds, burn, or infection	219,000
19.	Coronary artery bypass	191,000
20.	Pacemaker replacement, revision, or insertion	190,000
21.	Excision of intervertebral disc	188,000
22.	Myringotomy	187,000
23.	Closed reduction of fracture without internal fixation	183,000
24.	Bunion	182,000
25.	Placement or removal of internal fixation device without fracture reduction	173,000
26.	Partial excision of large intestine	169,000
27.	Arthroplasty of knee and ankle	161,000
28.	Total hip and/or arthroplasty of hip	159,000
29.	Repair of cystocele and rectocele	150,000
30.	Excision of semilunar cartilage of knee	147,000
31.	Local excision of tissue of bone	136,000
32.	Transurethral excision of bladder tissue	135,000
33.	Hemorrhoidectomy	129,000
34.	Free skin graft	120,000
35.	Mastectomy	116,000

THE INFLUENCE OF PHYSICIAN NUMBERS

An awareness of the past and present numbers of surgical operations allows manpower prognostication of physician numbers to evolve in a rational and pragmatic manner. Unfortunately, few manpower studies have utilized such information (15–21). Prior to 1970, little was known about surgical caseloads (22–23). In 1969, Lewis proposed a surgical variation of Parkinson's Law: "Patient admissions for surgery expand to fill beds, operating suites, and total surgical manpower" (24). A number of reports have noted large variations in the rates of surgical procedures internationally, nationally, and regionally (25–31). These and other studies propagated the concept that surgeons coming to a community perform surgery according to their own financial requirements (32–34).

My studies do not support this concept. If surgeons followed Parkinson's Law or truly practiced their craft in a capricious manner, then as the number of surgeons increases, the number of operations should correspondingly increase. However, this is not the case. Evidently, there are socioeconomic forces that do not allow a surgeon's scalpel to be wielded in an unbridled fashion. What are these and how have they come about?

Throughout the past five decades, health care planners have offered projections of the future need and supply of physicians in this nation. The first prominent such forecast was prepared in 1933 by Lee and Jones for the Committee on Cost of Medical Care of the American Medical Association (35). There followed the Ewing Report in 1948 (36), the Mountin-Pennel-Berger forecast in 1949 (37), the President's Commission on the Health Needs of the Nation in 1953 (38), the Bayne-Jones Report of 1958 (39), and the Bane Committee Report of 1959 (40), which appears to have furnished the foundation for the Health Professions Educational Assistance Act (P.L. 88-129) of 1963. This legislation established the first federal program that provided funds for medical education through grants for the construction of medical schools and loans to medical students. It was amended in 1965 (P.L. 28-290) to provide further monetary assistance.

Of all the reports that provide surgeons a glimpse into their own professional milieu, the *Study on Surgical Services for the United States* (SOSSUS) is the most well known (41). The report was commissioned by the American Surgical Association (ASA) and the American College of Surgeons (ACS) in 1969–70. It was a five-year effort that explored, among other topics, the organization, delivery, and financing of surgical services and surgical staffing.

Among the more interesting findings of SOSSUS was the remarkably low number of operations performed per surgeon on a yearly basis. Approximately 15 percent of board-certified surgical specialists carried out fewer than 50 operations a year, 31 percent between 100 and 199. Slightly over 33 percent performed 200 or more procedures. It was concluded that far too many physicians perform surgical operations and that the workloads of surgeons were much more modest than expected. It was suggested that the total volume of operations performed in this country could be handled by a substantially smaller cadre of board-certified surgeons. With this end in mind, the report made the following recommendations:

1. The number of training programs should be reduced and identified more closely with university centers as "affiliated hospitals."
2. The total number of persons entering practice with board certificates in general surgery and the surgical specialties should be reduced over the next ten years. . . . The total number of persons in training needs to be reduced and . . . tasks now performed by trainees [will] have to be assumed by other personnel.

SOSSUS's findings were corroborated by other studies. Hughes and others investigated workloads among general surgeons in a community practice and found them to be equivalent to only 4.3 hernia operations per week. Additional reports by Hughes demonstrated similar conclusions. This prompted his recommendation, closely paralleling SOSSUS's, that there appeared to be underutilization of costly and highly specialized surgical skills in this country. It was suggested that a diminution in the number of residents might result in increased efficiency in the delivery of surgical health care (42–44).

Following the publication of SOSSUS, proposals to place constraints on surgical staff numbers were widely heard (45–46). However, SOSSUS's recommendations were soon questioned by the American College of Surgeons. The accuracy of certain SOSSUS findings was challenged. As James Haug, director of the ACS's Department of Surgical Practice, wrote: "Unreliable data such as those cited [in SOSSUS] provide a poor basis for manpower estimates or for advanced planning" (47).

It was not unexpected that without ACS support SOSSUS would never achieve its intended impact on surgery in the United States. Six years after its publication, Williams showed SOSSUS's recommendations to have had no demonstrable effect; indeed, the surgeon population continued to grow (48). SOSSUS had become an orphan in the world of surgical politics.

The generally expansionist policies for physician numbers, recommended by medical staffing commissions and implemented by medical schools and state and federal government during the late 1960s and early 1970s, were beginning to have serious, unintended effects on the access to and the financing of health care (49). In 1965, there were 7,409 medical school graduates. By 1975, the number had increased to 12,714. The total continued to rise and in 1985 was 16,347. Current medical school enrollment has plateaued at approximately 17,000 first-year students. Clearly, government and society have managed to absorb increases in the physician population.

A controversy over whether the control of residency positions was an appropriate means of alleviating perceived specialty maldistribution was in part responsible for the passage of the Health Professions Educational Assistance Act of 1976 (P.L. 94-484). The law required medical schools to reserve primary-care residency positions in order to receive federal capitation grants.

Because of these and other concerns, the Graduate Medical Education National Advisory Committee (GMENAC) was chartered (April 1976) by the secretary of the Department of Health, Education, and Welfare to review residency training from the points of view of geographic and specialty distribution, as well as to oversee finance, entry procedures, examination, and foreign medical graduates. Of all the major reports on staffing numbers and needs, the GMENAC report is the most comprehensive and significant in terms of the possible consequences for medicine.

Published in 1980, the GMENAC report estimated a surplus of 38,600 surgeons in 1990: specifically, general surgeons, 11,800; obstetrician-gynecologic surgeons, 10,450; orthopedic surgeons, 5,000; ENT surgeons, 500; urologic surgeons, 1,650; ophthalmologic surgeons, 4,700; thoracic and cardiovascular surgeons, 850; neurosurgeons, 2,450; and plastic surgeons, 1,200 (50). To deal with this anticipated surplus, the following recommendations were made:

1. All medical schools should reduce entering class size in the aggregate by a minimum of 10 percent by 1984 relative to the 1978 enrollment.
2. To correct surpluses in a manner not disruptive to the graduate medical education system, no specialty should increase or decrease the number of first-year trainees in residency more than 20 percent by 1986, compared to 1979.
3. Medical school graduates in the 1980s should be strongly encouraged to enter those specialties where a shortage of physicians is expected.

Much criticism was directed at the GMENAC report and its methodology (51–52). However, the major findings could not be easily discounted. To add insult to injury, Williams, citing deficiencies in the report, recalculated the overall surplus of surgeons and found it to be 56,000 (53). The federal government clearly felt that the unprecedented numbers of physicians presented a problem for health care in this country.

Other warnings about surgeon surpluses were heard. Most notable was Dr. Francis Moore's: "By the year 2000, approximately two surgeons will be standing on the turf occupied by one surgeon in the years 1971 and 1972. The growth in the number of surgical specialists in this country is much faster than that of the population . . . and is rising quickly. . . . We believe that for surgery we will look and feel severely overcrowded. There is no escaping this fact" (54–58).

With the completion of the SOSSUS and GMENAC reports, it was possible to begin measuring their effects. To accomplish this, I reviewed the numbers of surgical residents on duty for the five-year period 1979–83 (59) and found that there was an increase of 7 percent of general surgeons, 3 percent of obstetricians-gynecologists, 11 percent of orthopedists, 1 percent of otolaryngologists, 2 percent of ophthalmologists, 5 percent of thoracic and cardiovascular surgeons, 19 percent of neurosurgeons, but a 3 percent decline of urologists. Essentially every specialty had more residents in 1983 than in 1979.

As with the SOSSUS report, no major surgical organization came forward to lend support to GMENAC's findings. Indeed, the *Bulletin of the American College of Surgeons* published a critique of the projections (60). As recently as June 1985, the Board of Regents of the ACS stated that "the College does not endorse any of the GMENAC recommendations regarding manpower because each one lacks a data base sufficiently firm and convincing to warrant acceptance by the College" (61).

Where does reality lie? Certain facts stand out. Numbers of surgical operations are increasing at less than 2 percent per year. When the growth of our population is taken into account, there has been an essential plateauing of the rates of surgical operations since 1975. This figure is contrasted to an ever-increasing supply of surgeons. In 1984, on average, a surgeon performed three operations per week.

Is a "manpower" crisis upon us? I believe it is just beginning. For the average surgeon, there are four years of medical school followed by five to seven years of graduate training. After residency programs, it usually takes three to five years to establish a practice and to have an impact on the surgical health care delivery system. Thus it takes between twelve and sixteen years to produce a well-trained surgeon. Surgeons who are beginning to influence the numbers of surgical procedures performed in 1987 would have graduated from medical school in the period 1971–75. If medical school enrollment did not reach its present levels until after 1975, surgeons trained in the past decade will not affect the health care system until after 1990. Therefore the adjustments required as the result of an increasing surgeon population will become considerably more imperative in the next decade and a half.

Critics of this scenario contend that recent federal legislative actions affecting foreign medical graduates will decrease the supply of physicians. However, this does not necessarily follow, since the American-born foreign medical graduate is rapidly replacing the foreign-born foreign medical graduate (62).

One major question remains. Why did an increasing rate of surgery suddenly plateau and, for some specialties, even decrease? One hypothesis is that for certain surgical specialties (general surgery, obstetrics-gynecology, ENT, and urology) an "optimum" level of surgical service was attained. Consequently, an increasing demand for their surgery was no longer present. Other specialties (vascular surgery, orthopedic surgery, ophthalmology, thoracic and cardiovascular surgery, neurosurgery) were strongly affected by electronic and other technologic advances. Since these innovations developed only over the last ten to twenty years, these specialties' "optimal levels" of surgical care were not reached by the mid-1970s. Unfortunately, it is difficult to define what the "optimum" level of surgical care should be for a given society (63–65).

The period in which the plateau occurred is concurrent with the initiation and expansion of the consumer movement in the United States. Some consumer groups have been especially vociferous in discussing the question of "unnecessary surgery" (66–69). Clearly, social forces can influence the utilization of surgical services and affect operation rates.

Some studies suggest that surgical rates are largely a function of broad political, economic, and other social forces (70). If this is true, then societal attempts to reduce medical expenditures and change the delivery system (e.g., health maintenance organizations, budget deficit reductions) will have an impact on our country's rate of surgery.

Within certain segments of organized surgery, some feel that there are not too many surgeons, but that too many "other" people (i.e., non–board certified and non–surgically trained physicians) are doing surgery (71). This position is quite tenuous considering the rapid and spectacular decline in the number of non–board certified surgeons in the United States (72). Nevertheless, any truth in this viewpoint should provide an even stronger stimulus to those who call for an elevation of surgical standards. As Moore (66) states:

we can hope that the voluntary national surgical organizations will see this [surgical surplus] as a realistic problem and face it squarely rather than adopting the juvenile view that surgeons are such wonderful people that one can never imagine a situation in which there are actually too many of them.

POLICY OPTIONS

I believe we face a surgical manpower crisis of unprecedented proportion (73–74). Accordingly, what situations may emerge from this surplus? Conceivably, by the year 2000, the average surgeon will be performing two or fewer surgical operations per week. This inability of the surgeon to find operation work can lead to several scenarios: (1) As surgeons perform fewer cases, their technical skills may decline, most notably for more complex operations. This may lead to increased morbidity and mortality. (2) Indications for surgical operations may become less stringent leading to more "unnecessary surgery." (3) Surgeons may be forced to practice more primary-care medicine to maintain their livelihood, further eroding their surgical skills.

The current direction might also produce two classes of surgeons: those who are splendid technicians and perform large numbers of operations and a dispirited and deprived group who complete little in the way of surgery and have a strong sense of disenfranchisement. All this points to a potentially crippling and tragic effect on the future quality of our country's surgical health care.

What can be done? The time has come for a conclave of clear-thinking and pragmatic surgeons to review the foundations on which surgery in the United States is built. The very fabric of our surgical education and training programs must be reevaluated.

1. Surgeons must acknowledge that a surgical surplus is present. They must be willing to accept the immensity of the problem and deal with it in a forthright and rational manner. Organized surgery, led by academic surgeons, must be at the forefront of this movement. The unwillingness of these surgeons to confront the problem has created many of the current difficulties.
2. The surgical community must actively begin to reduce the number of surgical residency positions. Non–university affiliated training centers should be brought under a university umbrella. Academic surgeons are the teachers of surgery. This position needs to be emphasized and strengthened.
3. It is imperative that departments of surgery in major teaching hospitals establish formal sections that have as their principal function

the responsibility for studying and carrying out research on the organization and delivery of surgical care. Forums for the discussion of socioeconomic problems must be provided at all national meetings, especially the ACS. Continued passivity will only lead to greater and perhaps unnecessary restrictions on the practice of surgery.

REFERENCES

1. Rutkow, I.M. Unnecessary surgery: What is it? *Surg Clin N Amer* 62:613–25 (1982).
2. McCarthy E.G., and Finkel, M. Surgical utilization in the U.S.A. *Med Care* 18:883–91 (1980).
3. Rutkow, I.M. *Surgical Health Care Delivery.* Philadelphia: W. B. Saunders Co. (1982).
4. Rutkow, I.M. Delivery of surgical health care in the United States. *Arch Surg* 116:963–69 (1981).
5. Rutkow, I.M. and Zuidema, G.D. "Unnecessary surgery": An update. *Surgery* 84:671–78 (1978).
6. Rutkow, I.M., and Zuidema, G.D. Surgical rates in the United States, 1966 to 1978. *Surgery* 89:151–62 (1981).
7. Vayda, E., Mindell, W.R., and Rutkow, I.M. A decade of surgery in Canada, England and Wales, and the United States. *Arch Surg* 117:846–53 (1982).
8. Rutkow, I.M. Rates of surgery in the United States: The decade of the 1970s. *Surg Clin N Amer* 62:559–78 (1982).
9. Rutkow, I.M., and Ernst, C.B. Vascular surgical manpower: Too much? Enough? Too little? Unknown? *Arch Surg* 117:1537–42 (1982).
10. Rutkow, I.M., and Starfield, B.H. Surgical decision making and operative rates. *Arch Surg* 119:899–905 (1984).
11. National Center for Health Statistics. *Development and Maintenance of a National Inventory of Hospitals and Institutions: Vital and Health Statistics.* PHS Pub. No. 1000- 1-3. Washington, D.C.: U.S. Government Printing Office (1965).
12. National Center for Health Statistics. *Detailed Diagnoses and Surgical Procedures for Patients Discharged from Short-stay Hospitals. United States, 1979.* DHHS (PHS) Pub No. 82-1274-1. Washington, D.C.: U.S. Government Printing Office (1982).
13. Detmer, D.E., and Buchanan-Davidson, D.J. Ambulatory surgery. *Surg Clin N Amer* 62:685–704 (1982).
14. Henderson, J. Surgicenters will mushroom if hospitals don't hobble growth. *Mod Hlthcare* 14:156–57 (1985).
15. Pearse, W.H., Mendenhall, R.C., Radecki, S.E., et al. Manpower for obstetrics-gynecology. 3: Contributions to total female medical care. *Am J Ob Gyn* 144:332–36 (1982).

16. Alford, B.R. Manpower needs in otorhinolaryngology. *Arch Oto* 104:725 (1978).
17. Fraley, E.E., and Watkins, E. Surgical and urologic manpower in the United States, 1969 to 1978. *J Urol* 127:218–23 (1982).
18. Worthen, D.M. Luxemberg, M.N., and Gutman, F.H. Ophthalmology manpower studies for the United States. Part 3: A survey of ophthalmologists' viewpoints and practice characteristics. *Ophthalmology* 88:45A–51A (1981).
19. Cleveland, R.J., Orthner, H.F., and Bahnson, H.T. Thoracic surgery manpower. The third manpower study of thoracic surgery: 1980 report of the ad hoc committee on manpower of the American Association for Thoracic Surgery and the Society of Thoracic Surgeons. *J Thor Card Surg* 84:921–32 (1982).
20. Watts, C. Neurosurgical manpower requirements for 1990: An estimate of the Graduate Medical Education National Advisory Committee. *Neurosurgery* 8:277–79 (1981).
21. O'Neil, J.A. Update on the analysis of the need for pediatric surgeons in the United States. *J Ped Surg* 15:918–24 (1980).
22. Collins, S.D. Frequency of surgical procedures among 9,000 families. *Pub Hlth Rep* 53:587–628 (1938).
23. Collins, S.D. Percentage of illnesses treated surgically among 9,000 families. *Pub Hlth Rep* 53:1593–1616 (1938).
24. Lewis, C.E. Variations in the incidence of surgery. *N Eng J Med* 281:880–85 (1969).
25. Bunker, J.P. Surgical manpower: A comparison of operations and surgeons in the United States and in England and Wales. *N Eng J Med* 282:135–41 (1970).
26. Vayda, E. A comparison of surgical rates in Canada and in England and Wales. *N Eng J Med* 289:1224–29 (1973).
27. Wennberg, E. and Gittelsohn, A.M. Small-area variations in health care delivery. *Science* 182:1102–5 (1973).
28. Wennberg, J.E. and Gittelsohn, A.M. Health care delivery in Maine: Patterns of use of common surgical procedures. *J Maine Med Assoc* 66:123–28 (1975).
29. Detmer, D.E. and Tyson, T.J. Regional differences in surgical care based upon uniform physician and hospital discharge-abstract data. *Ann Surg* 187:166–72 (1978).
30. McPherson, K., Wennberg, J.E., Hovind, O.B., and Clifford, P. Small-area variations in the use of common surgical procedures: An international comparison of New England, England, and Norway. *N Eng J Med* 307:1310–14 (1982).
31. Gittelsohn, A.M., and Wennberg, J.E. On the risk of organ loss. *J Chron Dis* 29:527–35 (1976).
32. Wilson, S.E., and Longmire, W.P. Does method of payment affect surgical care? *J Surg Res* 24:457–62 (1978).
33. LoGerfo, J.P., Efird, R.A., Diehr, P.K., and Richardson, W.C. Rates of sur-

gical care in prepaid group practices and the independent setting: What are the reasons for the differences? *Med Care* 17:1–11 (1979).
34. Chassin M.R., Brook, R.H., Park, R.E., et al. Variations in the use of medical and surgical services by the Medicare population. *N Eng J Med* 314:285–89 (1986).
35. Lee, R.I., and Jones, L.W. *The Fundamentals of Good Medical Care.* Chicago: University of Chicago Press (1933).
36. Ewing, O.R. *The National Health, a Ten-year Program: A report to the President.* Washington, D.C.: U.S. Government Printing Office (1948).
37. Mountin, J.W., Pennell, E.H., and Berger, A.G. *Health Service Areas: Estimates of Future Physician Requirements.* Public Health Bulletin No. 305. Washington, D.C.: U.S. Government Printing Office (1949).
38. President's Commission on the Health Needs of the Nation. *Building America's Health.* Vol. 2. Washington, D.C.: U.S. Government Printing Office (1953).
39. U.S. Department of Health, Education, and Welfare, Office of the Secretary. *The Advancement of Medical Research and Education through the Department of Health, Education, and Welfare. Final Report of the Secretary's Consultants on Medical Research and Education.* Washington, D.C.: U.S. Government Printing Office (1958). (Commonly referred to as the "Bayne-Jones Report".)
40. Bane, F. *Physicians for a Growing America.* Washington, D.C.: U.S. Government Printing Office (1959).
41. American College of Surgeons and the American Surgical Association. *Surgery in the United States: A Summary Report of the Study on Surgical Services in the United States (SOSSUS).* Chicago: American College of Surgeons (1975).
42. Hughes, E.F.X., Fuchs, V.R., Jacoby, J.E., and Lewit, E.M. Surgical workloads in a community practice. *Surgery* 71:315–23 (1972).
43. Hughes, E.F.X., Lewit, E.M., Watkins, R.N., and Handschin, R. Utilization of surgical manpower in a prepaid group practice. *N Eng J Med* 291:759–63 (1974).
44. Hughes, E.F.X., Lewit, E.M., and Lorenzo, F.V. Time utilization of a population of general surgeons in community practice. *Surgery* 77:371–77 (1975).
45. Moore, F.D., Zuidema, G.D., and Ballinger, W.F. Surgical manpower and public policy. *Surgery* 83:116–20 (1978).
46. Bloom, B.S., and Peterson, O.L. Changing the number of surgeons. *N Eng J Med* 303:1227–30 (1980).
47. Haug, J.N. Misconceptions on surgical residency positions. *Bull Amer Coll Surg* (1976).
48. Williams, D.C. Surgeons and Surgery in Rhode Island, 1970 and 1977. *N Eng J Med* 305:1319–23 (1981).
49. Bloom, B.S., and Peterson, O.L. Physician manpower expansionism: A policy review. *Ann Intern Med* 90:249–56 (1979).
50. *GMENAC Summary Report.* Vol. 1: *Report of the Graduate Medical Education National Advisory Committee to the Secretary, Department of*

Health and Human Services, United States Department of Health and Human Services. Washington, D.C.: U.S. Government Printing Office (1980).
51. McNutt, D.R. GMENAC: Its manpower forecasting framework. Am J Pub Hlth 71:1116–24 (1981).
52. Reinhardt, U.E. The GMENAC forecast: An alternative view. Am J Pub Hlth 71:1149–57 (1981).
53. Williams, D.C. Surgery and the GMENAC report: A reality test. Surgery 95:347–52 (1984).
54. Moore, F.D., Nickerson, R.J., Colton, T., et al. National surgical patterns as a basis for residency training plans: The response of a panel of surgeons. Arch Surg 112:125–47 (1977).
55. Moore, F.D. Surgical manpower: Past and present reality, estimates for 2000. Surg Clin N Amer 62:579–602 (1982).
56. Moore, F.D. A community-size model for physician distribution in the United States. J Clin Surg 1:162–73, 242–55 (1982).
57. Moore, F.D. Are there too many surgeons? In practice, or in training? Or neither, or both? In: Delaney, J.P., and Varco, R.L., eds., Controversies in Surgery, Vol. 2. Philadelphia: W.B. Saunders Co. (1983).
58. Moore, F.D. Medical and surgical manpower and economic phenomena. Surgery 95:374–75 (1984).
59. Eighty-fifth annual report on medical education in the United States, 1984–1985. JAMA 254:1567 (1985).
60. A critique of the GMENAC physician manpower projections for 1990. Bull Amer Coll Surg (1980).
61. American College of Surgeons. The American College of Surgeons in an Era of Societal Transformation. Chicago: American College of Surgeons (1985).
62. Stimmel, B. Medical students trained abroad and medical manpower: Recent trends and predictions. N Eng J Med 310:230–35 (1984).
63. Rutkow, I.M., Gittelsohn, A.M., and Zuidema, G.D. Surgical decision making: The reliability of clinical judgment. Ann Surg 190:409–19 (1979).
64. Rutkow, I.M. Surgical decision making: The reproducibility of clinical judgment. Arch Surg 117:337–40 (1982).
65. Rutkow, I.M. The reliability and reproducibility of the surgical decision-making process. Surg Clin N Amer 62:721–35 (1982).
66. Subcommittee on Oversight and Investigations of the Committee on Interstate and Foreign Commerce. Cost and Quality of Health Care: Unnecessary Surgery. Washington, D.C.: U.S. Government Printing Office (1976).
67. Subcommittee on Oversight and Investigations of the Committee on Interstate and Foreign Commerce. Report on Surgical Performance: Necessity and Quality. Washington, D.C.: U.S. Government Printing Office (1978).
68. Brody, J.E. Incompetent surgery is found not isolated. New York Times, January 27, 1976.
69. Denenberg, H.S. A shopper's guide to surgery. Conn Med 37:321–26 (1973).

70. Rutkow, I.M. The surgical decision-making process: Determinants of surgical rates. *Hlth Serv Res* 17:379–85 (1982).
71. Hanlon, C.R. Are there too many surgeons being trained? *In:* Delaney, J.P., and Varco, R.L., eds., *Controversies in Surgery,* vol. 2. Philadelphia: W.B. Saunders Co. (1983).
72. Moore, F.D., and Lang, S.M. Board-certified physicians in the United States. Specialty distribution and policy implications of trends during the past decade. *N Eng J Med* 304:1078–83 (1981).
73. Wangensteen, S.L. Changing prospects for the new surgical resident. *Am J Surg* 150:650–54 (1986).
74. Iglehart, J.K. The future supply of physicians. *N Eng J Med* 314:860–64 (1986).

3 Regional Variation in Surgical Procedures

Madelon Lubin Finkel, Ph.D.

Medicine is an art that is still very much dominated by different schools of thought in different parts of the country. Physicians are influenced by a complex interaction of concern for their patients, regard for the well-being of society, and their own self-interest (1). Studies have shown wide variations in many aspects of medical practice: hospital admissions, length of stay, surgical utilization, drug prescribing, and diagnostic test ordering. Physicians seem to render different types and amounts of medical care for patients with similar problems, even when the case mix and severity of illness are considered.

As the potential benefits, risks, and monetary costs of medical interventions have escalated, the choices made by physicians have a far greater impact on the individual patient and on society than before. Concomitantly, expanding diagnostic and therapeutic tools have made the selection of a correct strategy more complex and potentially more costly. Physicians are constantly faced with an increasing number of available options (2). Recent technological advances have facilitated a successful surgical outcome as well as complicated and intensified the work of those who are responsible for the process. Computerized tomography, ultrasound technology, cardiac catheterization, arteriography, nuclear magnetic resonance, and the introduction of laser therapy have revolutionized many surgical procedures and made possible the development of other surgical procedures that were deemed too risky or dangerous a few years ago.

The United States is a heterogeneous nation, and it is unrealistic to expect homogeneity in physician behavior or in pricing of services. Some variation is, in fact, understandable and appropriate; there are differences in patients' risks, signs, and symptoms. Thus some of the variations in practice patterns are unavoidable. However, regional and small-area variations noted by many researchers imply that other factors are contributing to differences in rates.

REGIONAL DIFFERENCES

Regional differences in hospital utilization rates across the country, known to be quite substantial, have been a focus of concern for some time. Three frequently mentioned explanations have been suggested:

1. The availability and organizational structure of health services determines hospital use (the Roemer hypothesis).
2. Physicians' styles of practice vary across regions.
3. The health needs of local populations vary from region to region.

Knickman and Foltz, in a well-designed study, found that the variation in hospital use between New York City and Los Angeles residents reflects variations in population characteristics (3). Their research provided a method for making quantitative estimates of utilization differences accounted for by several different population characteristics. They also found that organizational factors and physicians' style of practice may explain different admission rates and average lengths of stay. However, they caution that differences across areas are not the same as factors that explain differences across other units. While population characteristics play an important role, other variables such as physicians' practice styles, availability of alternative care, and reimbursement systems must be considered.

The literature has discussed at length the variation in clinical patterns across geographic boundaries and between practice settings. Small-area studies have shown variation in surgical procedures performed within and across areas. There is documentation of lower hospital utilization among those enrolled in HMOs and in other prepaid group practices as compared to those in conventional practice settings. There is wide variation reported in studies on the utilization patterns of acute-care hospital days, surgical procedures, and laboratory testing. While the evidence is convincing that differences exist, the reasons are not well understood.

Research shows that variations in practice patterns may occur primarily in the "gray areas" in which equally competent physicians disagree; that is, there is disagreement as to the preferred course of treatment (4). Hlatky, for example, found that identical patients had their medical problems evaluated and treated differently in different practice settings (5).

Chassin and others measured geographic differences in the use of medical and surgical services during 1981 among the Medicare population and found large geographic variations in the rates of many procedures. Of the 123 procedures studied, 67 had at least threefold differences between the highest and lowest rates. They found that individual areas did not exhibit highest or lowest rates with any consistency and that the variations could not have been due to the behavior of individual physicians. The researchers could not establish the "correct" rates for any given procedure. After they adjusted the rates for age and sex, the data showed that among those procedures exhibiting the greatest variations were injection of hemorrhoids, hip arthroplasty, arthrocentesis, mediastinoscopy and coronary artery bypass surgery. Among those procedures exhibiting the least variation were cholecystectomy, prostatectomy, lens extraction, inguinal hernia repair, and diagnostic upper gastrointestinal endoscopy.

It is often assumed in American society that more is always better. But the risk of a particular intervention may exceed the benefits. Overutilization can generate, not only unnecessary costs, but also unnecessary suffering. More is not always better. Nevertheless, underutilization can also generate substantial subsequent costs.

Persistent questions about the cost and medical appropriateness of surgery have given rise to several approaches to study surgical utilization.* The extent of unnecessary surgery has been a widely debated issue. The prevailing view is that from both a financial and medical perspective, the amount of "excessive" surgery is not trivial (7).

During the past two decades, much has been written about the propensity of Americans to undergo surgery (8–10). Studies have shown that overall surgical rates in the United States are considerably higher than those in other industrialized countries (11–13). Even within the United States, variations in surgical rates have been noted. Almost half a century ago, Glover showed the existence of considerable variation in tonsillectomy rates in various parts of England (14). He concluded that the differences in the incidence of this procedure were primarily due to professional judgment rather than to differences in morbidity. His thesis was that certain medical or surgical interventions could not be ascribed to medical diagnoses; they were a result of professional judgment, which differed from one physician to another.

In their landmark 1973 study, Wennberg and Gittelsohn documented sizable and persistent differences in the per capita rates of hospital admissions for surgical and other procedures among small areas (15). Other studies have focused on interregion and intraregion variations in surgical rates (16–23). The situation led some observers, including a congressional subcommittee, to suggest that unnecessary

---

*See, in particular, references 43 and 44 below.

surgery was being performed (24–27). The highly discretionary nature of medical care and the key role played by the physician in determining the nature and quantity of per capita consumption of medical services were emphasized.

More recently, McPherson and others examined the incidence of seven surgical procedures in small-area hospital service areas in Norway, England, and New England (27).* While the British and Norwegian rates were much lower than those for New England, domestic variation followed a characteristic pattern. Disagreements among clinicians seemed to influence practice patterns on both sides of the Atlantic. The procedures with little variation (appendectomy, hernia repair, cholecystectomy, for example) are those for which there is generally more physician consensus. Procedures for which there are alternative treatments or for which there is controversy over the diagnosis of the condition (hemorrhoidectomy, tonsillectomy, hysterectomy, and prostatectomy, for example) showed considerable variation. Roos and colleagues, too, found that Canadian physicians' discretion provided the best explanation for how surgical workloads change (28). Adjusting for case mix and controlling for physician specialty, they found that physicians who were high users of hospitals served 27 percent of the patients but that these patients consumed 42 percent of the hospital days.

In their report of variation in rates of utilization of surgical services in Massachusetts, Barnes and others also found twofold and threefold variations across geographic areas (29). They suggest that health care costs induced by high rates of utilization are substantial. Wennberg, McPherson, and Caper called for cost-containment programs based on fixed, per admission hospital prices (30). They argue that losses in hospital revenues due to the diagnosis-related groups (DRGs) payment system could be offset if physicians modified their admission policies.

Accepting the premise that variation exists and that its explanations are often not well understood, I focus here on trends in surgical procedures over time among the four geographic regions of the United States. I selected the decade from 1971 to 1982 specifically because during this time (1) there was an unprecedented rise in surgical rates, (2) health care costs soared and the hospital became the logical target of efforts to manage the health care dollar, (3) advances in medical technology and treatment procedures revolutionized the practice of medicine and surgery, and (4) focus on "overutilization" of specific procedures provided the impetus for the consumers of care to become more informed about health care and more involved in the containment of medical expenditures.

---

*See also chapter 1 above.

OVERALL TRENDS IN SURGICAL UTILIZATION

Surgical utilization rates as cited have been compiled by the National Center for Health Statistics (NCHS). Statistics are presented on surgical operations and procedures performed in nonfederal short-stay hospitals based on data abstracted by the Hospital Discharge Survey from a national sample of hospital records of discharged patients. Through a system of weighting measures, the data reflect unbiased national estimates of the absolute number of operations performed in any given year.

Until the early 1970s, the rate of surgery in the United States was fairly stable and consistent with population growth. Since 1971, however, it has grown rapidly. The rate of all operations performed per 100,000 people was 7,735 in 1965, compared to 7,805.3 in 1971. From 1971 to 1982, the rate steadily increased to 11,234.8, an increase of almost 44 percent.

Analysis of procedure-specific surgical rates clearly shows steady growth during this decade. In some cases, unparalleled growth occurred, for example, in coronary artery bypass (increased 532.4 percent), lens extraction (increased 119.7 percent), and cesarean section (increased 231.3 percent). Tonsillectomy and/or adenoidectomy was the only procedure to show a steady decline in the rate (decreased 59.6 percent).

Table 3.1 depicts surgical rates for some of the most commonly selected procedures performed in the United States for 1971 and 1982. The data clearly show marked increases for almost all procedures for each age group and for both sexes. There has been a very slight increase, for example, in the rate of hysterectomies performed from 1971 to 1982 (1.7 percent). The rate actually declined among those forty-five to sixty-four years old. In fact, the number and rate of hysterectomies peaked in 1975. The rate of vertebral surgery, too, declined among those older than sixty-five from 1971 to 1982 (see also chap. 2 above).

From 1971 to 1982, rates of total surgical procedures for males increased 44.5 percent; among females, the increase was 54.1 percent. The increase among the female population can be attributed to the increase in gynecological surgery, particularly for sterilization. During this decade, there has been a surge in the number of women electing surgical sterilization.

When the data are analyzed by age, the statistics show that surgery is performed more frequently with advancing age. Whereas there was a 22.7 percent increase in total surgical rates among those forty-five to sixty-four years old from 1971 to 1982, there was a 67.9 percent increase among those sixty-five and older during the same time period. In

TABLE 3.1. Rates per 100,000 Selected Surgical Procedures Analyzed by Age and Sex, 1971 and 1982

Procedure	45–64 Years		≥ 65 Years		Male		Female	
	1971	1982	1971	1982	1971	1982	1971	1982
Cholecystectomy	346.1	374.0	439.2	514.2	87.0	118.8	270.6	303.4
Coronary bypass	45.4	237.3	5.1	186.6	20.2	112.9	3.8	37.7
Excision of intervertebral cartilage and spinal fusion	155.2	190.7	112.4	61.5	100.2	113.3	56.6	84.8
Excision of semilunar cartilage and meniscus	57.3	86.6	15.3	46.9	76.9	102.8	22.6	37.7
Extraction of lens	152.8	256.9	873.4	1,707.7	101.2	207.1	134.8	310.5
Hysterectomy	491.8	408.4	148.1	216.6	N/A	N/A	537.5	546.7
Prostatectomy	133.7	216.3	761.0	974.8	209.5	332.9	N/A	N/A
Total operations performed	9,769.4	11,985.4	12,850.3	21,576.3	6,333.4	9,151.0	9,151.0	14,099.5

their study analyzing more than two million hospital discharges between 1972 and 1981, Valvona and Sloan found that surgical admissions of patients sixty-five and older increased 106 percent during the last decade as compared to 46 percent for surgical patients overall (31). Much of the increase can be traced to new or improved surgical procedures. For example, coronary artery bypass surgery increased more for elderly patients, as did lens extraction and hysterectomies.

As life expectancy continues to increase, the number of elderly (65–84 years) and the very old (older than 85) will continue to increase. The implications of these increases are great, as the elderly have more hospitalizations and more disabilities than their younger counterparts. Therefore it is expected that surgery rates for this cohort will continue to increase steadily over time.

REGIONAL VARIATIONS IN SURGICAL RATES

Statistics from 1971 to 1982 show that the rates of patient discharges with surgery increased steadily for each of the four regions of the country. Tables 3.2–3.6 show selected surgical rates by region for 1971 and 1982. The overall increase from 1971 to 1982 ranged from 59 percent in the South to 21.1 percent in the Northeast. The following discussion focuses on the specific procedures highlighted for analysis.

Cesarean Section

The magnitude of C-section rates in the United States has been of increasing public concern. Reasons for escalating rates continue to be the subject of much controversy and study. Explanations offered have included fear of litigation, a disproportionate number of repeat C-sections, and changes in the management of certain high-risk or difficult births. A consensus development conference held in 1980 formulated recommendations that were expected to lead to a decrease in national cesarean section rates. Contrary to expectations, a continuing increase in the rates has been evident (33).

Nationwide, the rate of C-sections increased almost 120 percent from 1971 to 1982. There were huge regional differences in the rate of increase during this time period: up 133.8 percent in the Northeast, up 192.4 percent in the North Central region, up 353.2 percent in the South, and up 267.1 percent in the West. One could conjecture that the differences in the rates reflect different philosophies among obstetricians across the country.

In addition to regional variations in the rates, charges for C-sec-

TABLE 3.2. Selected Surgical Rates per 100,000 People by Region, 1971 and 1982 (Total U.S.)

Procedures	1971	1982	% Change 1971–1982
C-section	95.9	317.7	+119.7
Cholecystectomy	182.1	214.3	+17.7
Coronary bypass	11.7	74.0	+532.4
Excision of intervertebral cartilage and spinal fusion	77.6	98.6	+27.1
Excision of semi-lunar cartilage	49.3	65.5	+32.9
Extraction of lens	118.6	260.6	+119.7
Hysterectomy	278.2	282.8	+1.7
Prostatectomy	101.0	155.9	+54.4
Tonsillectomy and/or andenoidectomy	472.0	190.7	−59.6
Total operations performed*	7,805.3	11,234.8	+43.9

*Excluding non-surgical procedures

TABLE 3.3. Selected Surgical Rates per 100,000 People by Region, 1971 and 1982 (Northeast)

Procedures	1971	1982	% Change 1971–1982
C-section	122.1	285.5	+133.8
Cholecystectomy	219.2	208.7	−4.8
Coronary bypass	6.1	46.3	+659.0
Excision of intervertebral cartilage and spinal fusion	67.6	55.6	−17.8
Excision of semi-lunar cartilage	47.1	55.3	+17.4
Extraction of lens	125.0	223.6	+78.9
Hysterectomy	262.2	197.9	−24.5
Prostatectomy	116.8	161.0	+37.8
Tonsillectomy and/or andenoidectomy	397.4	131.1	−67.0
Total operations performed*	8,614.8	10,435.9	+21.1

*Excluding non-surgical procedures

TABLE 3.4. Selected Surgical Rates per 100,000 People by Region, 1971 and 1982 (North Central)

Procedures	1971	1982	% Change 1971–1982
C-section	96.3	281.6	+192.4
Cholecystectomy	214.9	232.4	+8.1
Coronary bypass	19.5	90.2	+362.6
Excision of intervertebral cartilage and spinal fusion	87.0	119.9	+37.8
Excision of semilunar cartilage	55.1	79.1	+43.6
Extraction of lens	138.5	316.5	+128.5
Hysterectomy	287.7	286.6	−0.4
Prostatectomy	122.5	174.2	+42.2
Tonsillectomy and/or andenoidectomy	603.8	274.8	−54.5
Total operations performed*	8,848.3	13,116.4	+48.2

*Excluding non-surgical procedures

TABLE 3.5. Selected Surgical Rates per 100,000 People by Region, 1971 and 1982 (South)

Procedures	1971	1982	% Change 1971–1982
C-section	82.5	373.9	+353.2
Cholecystectomy	152.3	218.8	+43.7
Coronary bypass	9.6	74.2	+672.9
Excision of intervertebral cartilage and spinal fusion	81.8	102.9	+25.8
Excision of semi-lunar cartilage	41.7	54.8	+31.4
Extraction of lens	99.4	211.0	+112.3
Hysterectomy	290.2	347.3	+19.7
Prostatectomy	78.6	140.8	+79.1
Tonsillectomy and/or andenoidectomy	428.0	167.8	−60.8
Total operations performed*	6,814.3	10,834.4	+59.0

*Excluding non-surgical procedures

TABLE 3.6. Selected Surgical Rates per 100,000 People by Region, 1971 and 1982 (West)

Procedures	1971	1982	% Change 1971–1982
C-section	82.7	303.6	+267.1
Cholecystectomy	144.6	188.5	+30.4
Coronary bypass	11.6	83.0	+615.5
Excision of intervertebral cartilage and spinal fusion	78.1	110.5	+41.5
Excision of semi-lunar cartilage	60.7	77.4	+27.5
Extraction of lens	121.4	313.8	+158.5
Hysterectomy	283.4	259.8	−10.8
Prostatectomy	92.5	152.2	+64.5
Tonsillectomy and/or andenoidectomy	477.1	185.5	−61.1
Total operations performed*	6,752.1	10,330.1	+53.0

*Excluding non-surgical procedures

tions (approximately twice that of vaginal deliveries) vary considerably. The average total cost of a cesarean in the United States is $4,130 (hospital and physician charges). Lowest costs were reported in the South Central states (Arkansas, Kentucky, and Mississippi), while the highest costs were reported in California and New York.

Average physician charges total $1,270, with physicians in California and New York charging the highest rates ($1,890 and $1,780, respectively) and physicians in Iowa charging the least ($910) (34).

Cholecystectomy

Removal of the gall bladder is one of the most common interabdominal procedures in general surgery. The procedure is performed more frequently on women, and the average age of most patients is the mid-forties. Stones in the gall bladder will develop in approximately 20 percent of all Americans over the age of forty. Many will remain asymptomatic; therefore, the presence of stones is not the only prerequisite for a cholecystectomy. Conservative treatments are available, noninvasive treatments are available, and less complicated surgeries are viable alternatives to the more costly cholecystectomy.

Regional variations in the rate of cholecystectomies performed from 1971 to 1982 are striking. Whereas nationwide the rate increased almost 18 percent, in the Northeast it actually declined by 4.8 percent. In the North Central region the rate increased 8.1 percent, but in the South and West the rate soared 43.7 percent and 30.4 percent respectively. Not only do cholecystectomy rates differ by geographic area, but the average charges also vary. The highest average total cost was in the Pacific region ($6,740, which is 224 percent above the national average), and the lowest in the East South Central region ($5,020, or 8 percent below the national average).

While explanations for these discrepancies are unclear, it can be said that in some regions of the country, some unnecessary surgery is being performed.

Coronary Bypass Surgery

The growth in the number and rate of coronary artery bypass operations has been spectacular during the 1970s. New technological advances have made the procedure one of the most frequently performed among those forty-five to sixty-four as well as those over sixty-five. Nationwide, the rate increased 532.4 percent from 1971 to 1982. With the exception of the North Central region, the rate increased well over 600 percent; it increased 362.6 percent in the North Central region.

However, nonsurgical treatment for severe heart disease has improved to the point where drugs and diet programs can be as effective as the surgery in many patients. "Flunking" a treadmill exercise test for heart disease is not sufficient reason to send a patient for coronary artery bypass surgery. Percutaneous transluminal angioplasty, too, is an effective means of relieving the obstructions that produce the chest discomfort of angina. Surgical treatment or lifelong medical management must be determined by evaluating the patient's medical symptoms and life style. While neither treatment cures the disease, one may offer more effective rehabilitation and prolongation of life.

Coronary artery bypass surgery is one of the most costly, and variations in charges have been noted across the country. The average cost, including hospital charges and surgical and physician fees, is

$21,800 (1985 dollars). California had the highest charge ($30,800), and Kentucky the lowest ($13,500) (35). According to a Metropolitan Life Insurance report, price differences are primarily a result of varying costs of living. Given the complexity of the procedure and the costs associated with it, it might be more prudent to designate regional centers for this type of surgery since frequency of performing the operation and mortality have been correlated.

Surgery on the Back

Excision of intervertebral cartilage and spinal fusion are procedures highly dependent on surgeon judgment and discretion. As a result of different philosophies, variations in the rates are expected. Nationwide, from 1971 to 1982, the rate increased 27.1 percent. However, data not presented showed a steady decline in the rate from 1978 to 1981. For some unexplained reason, the rate jumped almost 20 percent from 1981 to 1982. Perhaps the change in ICDA coding has affected the statistics since there was a dramatic shift in codes from the ICDA-8 to ICDA-9 revision.

In the Northeast, there has been a steady decline in the rate from 1971 to 1982 (down 16.8 percent), but in the North Central region, there was a healthy 37.8 percent increase in the rate during the same time period. There was a 25.8 percent increase in the rate in the South and a 41.5 percent increase in the West during the past decade.

Surgery on the Knee

A complete tear of the anterior cruciate ligament represents the beginning of a continuum of functional disability. However, there are conflicting opinions on the degree of disability associated with the anterior cruciate ligament syndrome; there is no agreement in the literature as to what constitutes a significant symptom. There is also debate about the indications for nonsurgical treatment or for acute surgical repair and augmentation (36).

Medical technology has affected dramatically the way orthopedists diagnose and treat knees and, to a lesser extent, other joints. Microsurgery has revolutionized treatment of damaged tissue without having to open up the knee capsule. For a decade, this diagnostic and mini-operative technique had been virtually ignored by most orthopedic surgeons. Today, with more than 600,000 arthroscopic procedures performed each year in the United States, some orthopedists feel that there is a tendency to overuse arthroscopy. The statistics presented do not reflect the growth in arthroscopic surgery of the knee; rather, they illustrate the trend in the number of meniscectomies performed.

Nationwide, the rate of meniscectomies increased 32.9 percent from 1971 to 1982. While the Northeast showed the smallest increase (17.4 percent) and the North Central region the highest (43.6 percent), the Southern and Western regions showed increases fairly consistent with the national rate over time (31.4 percent and 27.5 percent, respectively). These statistics clearly reflect differences of opinion regarding the need and appropriateness of surgery on the knee.

Excision of the Lens

Cataract surgery is one of the most safe and effective major operations being performed today. Advances in surgical techniques and in the design and manufacture of the artificial intraocular lens have permitted the procedures to be performed on an outpatient basis. As a result, cataract surgery has become a booming business in the United States. Billions of dollars are spent on the removal of cataracts and the implantation of intraocular lenses. While one would have thought that outpatient surgery would have saved millions of dollars, a two-year study sponsored by the House Select Committee on Aging revealed that almost half of the annual bill to Medicare for cataract surgery is lost to fraud, waste, and abuse. It was noted that Medicare paid several times the inpatient rate for outpatient surgery (37). The blame for the abuses can be placed on certain manufacturers, ophthalmologists, and officials in the federal government who have failed to correct wasteful and illogical practices.

The rate for this procedure increased 68 percent among those forty-five to sixty-four years of age from 1971 to 1982 and almost 96 percent among those over sixty-five years. Nationwide, the rate increased almost 120 percent for all ages. In the Northeast, the rate increased 78.9 percent; in the North Central region, 128.5 percent. In the South, the rate increased 112.3 percent, but in the West, where many retirement communities are located, the rate soared 158.5 percent. If one were to analyze the data by state, Florida, Arizona, and California would show highest rates primarily because of the large numbers of elderly patients residing there.

Hysterectomy

Hysterectomies are one of the most commonly performed major operations in the United States. The rates have fluctuated over the years: 278.2 per 100,000 people in 1971, 301.1 per 100,000 people in 1978, and 295.5 per 100,000 in 1981. In 1982, the rate was 282.8 per 100,000 people, a 1.7 percent increase from 1971.

TABLE 3.7. Number of Hysterectomies Performed by Region in Selected Years

Region	Number per 100,000 People				% Change 1971–1982
	1971	1978	1981	1982	
Northeast	262.2	204.9	199.1	197.9	−24.5
North Central	287.7	317.2	287.7	286.6	−0.4
South	290.2	372.3	352.3	347.3	+19.7
West	283.4	250.3	314.1	259.8	−10.8

Regionally, the rates have varied tremendously (see table 3.7). These variations leave open the question of what rate is appropriate. Are too many hysterectomies being performed in the South and too few in the Northeast? Not only do the rates vary, but the costs of the procedure varies dramatically. The average total charge for a hysterectomy in the United States was $4,710 in 1983. In the states of California and Florida, the average costs were more than $4,000, while in the state of Kentucky, the average cost was $2,500 (38).

Barnes, in his analysis of over 19,000 hysterectomies in three Northeastern states, found that more than 92 percent were performed for indications other than malignant diseases, sepsis, or immediate complications of pregnancy (38). While sterilization or menstrual disorders may be a major consideration in the decision to perform the operation, there certainly are less drastic and less costly ways to achieve the same or similar results.

Surgery on the Prostate

Transurethral resection of the prostate is generally regarded as the best treatment for symptomatic benign prostatic hypertrophy in all but the largest glands. Surgery on the prostate has increased 54.4 percent from 1971 to 1982. Among those forty-five to sixty-four years old, there was a 61.8 percent increase during this time period, while among those over sixty-five, there was a 28 percent increase.

In the two regions of the country where there are more retirees, the increase was the greatest (79.1 percent in the South and 64.5 percent in the West). In the Northeast, the rate increased almost 38 percent, and in the North Central region, 42.2 percent.

Tonsil and Adenoid Surgery

The removal of the tonsils and adenoids is one of the few surgical procedures to exhibit a steady decline over time. Indications for surgery have been modified, and this is indicative of the decision not to operate. It is now generally agreed that children with repeated episodes of tonsillitis do not qualify as an absolute candidate for surgery. Decision for surgery should be based on a number of specific episodes of tonsillitis as well as on the total picture that the child presents over a period of time. The child should be evaluated for allergies, sinusitis, cystic fibrosis, or any other defects to determine whether the problem of recurrent upper respiratory infection and sore throats can be handled in a nonsurgical manner (40). From 1971 to 1982, the rate declined almost 60 percent. Each region of the country showed a decline in the rate over time, and the rates for each are remarkably similar.

COMMENTARY

Although the explanations for the rise in surgical utilization and the variations among regions are by no means clear, the statistics do show the need to investigate and to understand the phenomenon. Perhaps John Bunker's suggestion that surgical demand will increase as the public becomes more fully informed is materializing (40). Certainly the number of surgeons has been shown to have a powerful effect on the rate of surgery (see chap. 2). The greater comprehensiveness of health insurance coverage, the availability of Medicare, hospital reimbursement practices, and advances in technology also contribute to the increase, but to what extent is not clear.

While the explanations for the increases are not obvious, there is no question that the various surgical subspecialties must be individually analyzed before generalizations can be made. There have been widespread charges and insinuations about the performance of large numbers of "unjustified" operations. The lack of an acceptable definition as to what unnecessary surgery really is confounds the issue. Treatment styles change over time and within geographic areas; differences among surgeons regarding surgical versus nonsurgical treatments exist. For most conditions, the efficacy of either surgical or nonsurgical treatment has not been firmly established. Thus, some researchers feel that the issue of unnecessary surgery will not be resolved until the question of efficacy of various treatments is answered (42).

Patterns of high, moderate, or low rates for medical care within a community tend to reflect the preferences and practice styles of local physicians and surgeons. Low-variation admissions tend to be those for which the condition is clearly identified and for which there is professional consensus about a particular treatment.

In the long run, improvement in medical decisions depends upon reducing the uncertainties physicians and patients face in deciding on the use of specific treatments. In the short run, feedback on geographic variations, especially on high variations, can be an effective tool for reducing the use of hospitals without jeopardizing the access to and the quality of care (43).

REFERENCES

1. Eisenberg, J. Physician Utilization: The state of research about physicians' practice patterns. *Med Care* 23:461–83 (1985).
2. Doubilet, P., and McNeal, B. Clinical decision-making. *Med Care* 23:648–62 (1985).
3. Knickman, J., and Foltz, A. Regional differences in hospital utilization. *Med Care* 22:971–84 (1984).
4. Luft, H. Variations in clinical practice patterns. *Arch Intern Med* 143:1861–62 (1983).
5. Hlatky, M., Lee, K., Botvinik, E., and Brundage, B. Diagnostic test use in different practice settings. *Arch Intern Med* 143:1886–89 (1983).
6. Chassin, M.R., Brook, R.H., Park, R.E., et al. Variations in the use of medical and surgical services by the Medicare population. *N Eng J Med* 314:285–89 (1986).
7. Brook, R.H., and Lohr, K.N., Second-opinion programs: Beyond cost-benefit analyses. *Med Care* 20:1–2 (1982).
8. McCarthy, E.G., and Finkel, M.L. Surgical utilization in the U.S.A. *Med Care* 18:883–92 (1980).
9. Rutkow, I.M., and Zuidema, G.D. Surgical rates in the United States, 1966 to 1978. *Surgery* 89:151–62 (1981).
10. Rutkow, I.M. Rates of surgery in the United States: The decade of the 1970s. *Surg Clin N Amer* 62:559–78 (1982).
11. Pearson, R.J.C., Smedby, B., Berfenstam, R., et al. Hospital caseloads in Liverpool, New England, and Uppsala: An international comparison. *Lancet* 2:559–66 (1968).
12. Bunker, J.P. Surgical manpower: A comparison of operations and surgeons in the United States and in England and Wales. *N Eng J Med* 282:135–44 (1970).
13. Vayda, E., Mindell, W.R., and Rutkow, I.M. A decade of surgery in Canada, England and Wales, and the United States. *Arch Surg* 117:846–53 (1982).
14. Glover, J.A. The incidence of tonsillectomy in school children. *Proc Roy Soc Med* 31:95–112 (1938).
15. Wennberg, J.E., and Gittelsohn, A.M. Small-area variations in health care delivery. *Science* 182:1102–8 (1973).
16. Bunker, J.P., Barnes, B.A., and Mosteller, F., eds., *Costs, Risks, and Benefits of Surgery*. New York: Oxford University Press (1977).
17. Detmer, D.E., and Tyson, T.J. Regional differences in surgical care based upon uniform physician and hospital discharge-abstract data. *Ann Surg* 187:166–69 (1978).
18. Taylor, J.M. Medicare payments and changes in the rate of cataract extraction. *Ophthalmology.* 88:41A–46A (1981).

19. Walker, A.M., and Jick, H. Temporal and regional variation in hysterectomy rates in the United States, 1970–1975. *Am J Epi* 110:41–51.
20. Vayda, E., and Mindell, W.R. Variations in operative rates: What do they mean? *Surg Clin N Amer* 62:627–39 (1982).
21. Roos, N.P. Hysterectomy: Variations in rates across small areas and across physicians' practices. *Am J Pub Hlth* 74:327–35 (1984).
22. Roos, N.P., and Roos, L.L. Surgical rate variations: Do they reflect the health or socioeconomic characteristics of the population. *Med Care* 20:945–58 (1982).
23. Rutkow, I.M., and Zuidema, G.D. Unnecessary surgery: An update. *Surgery* 84:671–78 (1978).
24. Schlicke, C.P. Doctor, is this operation necessary? *Am J Surg* 134:3–12 (1977).
25. Paulshock, B.Z. Unnecessary surgery: Who'll have the final say? *Med Econ* 54:75–80 (1977).
26. Subcommittee on Oversight and Investigation. *Cost and Quality of Health Care: Unnecessary Surgery.* Washington, D.C.: U.S. Government Printing Office (1976).
27. McPherson, K., Wennberg, J.E., Hovind, O.B., et al. Small-area variations in the use of common surgical procedures: An international comparison of New England, England, and Norway. *N Eng J Med* 307:1310–14 (1982).
28. Roos, N., Flowerden, G., Wajda, A., et al. Variations in physicians' hospitalization practices: A population-based study in Manitoba, Canada. *Am J Pub Hlth* 76:45–51 (1986).
29. Barnes, B.A., O'Brien, E., Comstock, C., et al. Report on variation in rates of utilization of surgical services in the Commonwealth of Massachusetts. *JAMA* 254:371–75 (1985).
30. Wennberg, J.E., McPherson, K., and Caper, P. Will payment based on diagnosis-related groups control hospital costs? *N Eng J Med* 311:295–300 (1984).
31. Valvona, J., and Sloan, F.A. Rising surgical rates among the elderly. *Health Affairs* 4:108–19 (1985).
32. Gleicher, N. Cesarean section rates in the United States. *JAMA* 252:3273–76 (1984).
33. Metropolitan Life Insurance Co. *Statistical Bulletins.* July/Sept. 1986.
34. Metropolitan Life Insurance Co. *Statistical Bulletin.* April/June 1986.
35. Noyes, F.R., and McGinniss, G.H. Controversy about treatment of the knee with anterior cruciate laxity. *Clin Orthop* 198:61–76 (1985).
36. Pepper, C. Abuses surrounding cataract industry call for public policy reforms. *Business and Health* 4:58–59 (1986).
37. Metropolitan Life Insurance Co. *Statistical Bulletin.* July/Sept. 1985.
38. Barnes, B.A. An overview of hospital gynecologic pactice. *Primary Care* 8:165 (1981).
39. Sprinkle, P.M., Sorensen, H., Hellerstein, S., et al. Tonsillectomies and adenoidectomies. *In:* Jazbi, B., ed. *The Otolaryngologic Clinics of North America* 10:245–47 (1977).

40. Bunker, J.P., and Brown, B.W. The physician-patient as informed consumer of surgical services. *N Eng J Med* 290:1051 (1974).
41. Vayda, E., and Mindell, W.R. Variations in operative rates: What do they mean? *In:* Rutkow, I.M., ed., Surgical health care delivery. *Surg Clin N Amer* 62:627–40 (1982).
42. Caper, P., Keller, R., and Rohlf, P. Teaching physician practice patterns for quality care. *Business and Health* 3:7–9 (1986).
43. Zuidema, G.D., ed. *Surgery in the United States: A Summary Report of the Study of Surgical Services for the United States.* Chicago: R.R. Donnelly and Sons (1975).
44. Rutkow, I.M., ed. *Surg Clin N Amer* 62, 4 (1982).

4 Variation in Surgical Practice: A Proposal for Action

John Wennberg, M.D.

Most people view the medical care they receive as a necessity provided by doctors who adhere to scientific norms based on previously tested and proven treatments. When the contents of the medical care "black box" are examined more closely, however, the type of medical service provided is often found to be as strongly influenced by subjective factors related to the attitudes of individual physicians as it is by science. These subjective considerations, which I call collectively the "practice style factor," can play a decisive role in determining what specific services are provided a given patient as well as whether the treatment occurs in the ambulatory or the inpatient setting. As a consequence, this style factor has profound implications for the patient and the payer of care.

For example, the practice style factor affects whether patients with menopausal symptoms, with hypertrophy of the tonsil, with hyperplasia of the prostate, with mild angina, or with a host of other ailments receive conservative treatments in an ambulatory setting or undergo a surgical operation in a hospital. It also affects whether patients with relatively minor medical conditions such as bronchitis or gastroenteritis or who need minor surgical procedures such as cystoscopy, teeth extractions, sterilization, or breast biopsy receive their care in a hospital or elsewhere. The practice style that favors inpatient treatment greatly affects the demand for hospital care and has serious implications for efforts to constrain costs.

These implications become clear when one recognizes that, within a region or state, different opinions held by physicians concerning the need for hospitalization—as measured by per capita admission rates—are the most important determinant of variations in per capita costs for the treatment of specific diseases (1–4).* The different opinions of

---

This chapter is reprinted, in part, with permission from *Health Affairs* 6: (1984):6–32.

*This is a consistent finding, first reported for Vermont and Maine hospital markets and later confirmed for markets in Massachusetts, Iowa, and Michigan.

doctors over the need to hospitalize are much more influential in established total costs than differences in cost per case or the length of an inpatient stay.

Some of the differences in opinion arise because the necessary scientific information on outcomes is missing: controversies about alternative therapies cannot be resolved through appeal to existing evidence. To resolve the differences in opinion—and to learn whether high or low rates of admission reflect appropriate care—more scientific information must be obtained.

For other conditions, the practice style factor appears unrelated to scientific controversies. Physicians in some hospital markets practice medicine in ways that have extremely adverse implications for the cost of care, motivated perhaps by reasons of their own or their patients' convenience, or because of individualistic interpretations of the requirements for "defensive medicine." Whatever the reason, it certainly is not because of adherence to medical standards based on clinical outcome criteria or even on statistical norms based on average performance. In some markets, a substantial proportion of hospitalizations are for cases that in other markets are usually treated outside the hospital. If more conservative, ambulatory-oriented practice styles were substituted—and if hospital administrators and trustees translated the decreased demand for hospital resources into a reduction in the capacity of the hospital industry—then substantial cost savings and improvements in quality could be realized without fear that needed services were being withheld.*

In this chapter, I propose a plan for dealing with the implications of variations in medical practice for health care outcome and cost containment. My goal is not to obliterate all variation from the practice of medicine. Obviously, physicians must have freedom to apply the skills of their profession as they and their patients see fit; after all, medicine remains as much art as science. Moreover, any enterprise as large as medical care will produce variations in approach. My targets are variations that are both substantial and reflective of supply factors rather than of scientific knowledge and the values, needs, or wants of patients.

My plan has three parts. The first calls for a closer monitoring of medical practice in local hospital markets, using epidemiologic techniques to obtain population-based measures of resource allocation, service use, and outcomes of health care. This information should be made available on a continuous basis to interested parties. Second, I recommend that the medical community and qualified researchers address

---

*Improvements in quality of care would follow a reduction in unnecessary hospitalizations, particularly for children and the elderly.

unanswered questions concerning the effectiveness of many common therapeutic interventions. The overriding questions in this regard are whether such interventions have beneficial outcomes and are relatively safe.

Third, I recommend that the medical community make greater efforts to deal with the cost-containment problem by reducing the use of hospitals for marginally indicated conditions, as may be determined from the monitoring of medical practice called for above. The challenge would be to translate these reductions in inpatient demand into reductions in the capacity of the hospital industry as a step toward moderating the growth of per capita health costs.

In advancing this plan, I draw on my experience with monitoring the performance of the medical care systems in New England over the past decade and, more recently, in Iowa. In these areas, I have worked closely with doctors and state medical societies to feed back to physicians the information I found. Their positive response to this information suggests that doctors and their professional organizations in other areas can be expected to assume leadership roles in projects that deal with the implications of the variation phenomenon for cost and medical outcome. But the feasibility of the plan will depend ultimately upon broad-based support from the private and public sector, including government. I offer some specific suggestions on the nature of that involvement.

EXAMINING THE "BLACK BOX" OF MEDICAL CARE

Before discussing my plan, I want to review the evidence that argues for attaching importance to supply factors in determining the demand for hospitalization. I also want to examine the variation phenomenon in greater detail, particularly its implications for cost containment.

Why is it that the norms of medical practice can be so loose or ambiguous as to allow a wide range of professional discretion? The answer is seen in a review of the medical literature on the degree of professional consensus concerning the value of specific treatments and in the critical examination of the scientific strengths and weaknesses of the studies that support a particular viewpoint.

The procedures exhibiting the most variation are often for conditions that are part of the aging process. The controversies arise because for such conditions the natural history of the untreated or conservatively treated case is often poorly understood, and well-designed clinical trials are notably absent. Examples include hysterectomy for noncancerous conditions, prostatectomy for benign hyperplasia of the prostate, tonsillectomy for hypertrophy of the tonsil, and coronary bypass surgery for mild angina. Well-defined scientific norms simply do not exist to limit the options physicians select to treat these maladies. As a consequence, the opinions of individual doctors can vary substantially, based upon subjective experience. Because many of the conditions are associated with aging, the number of candidates that could qualify for operative intervention is sometimes upwardly limited only by the size of the population.

For example, I have observed that in Maine, by the time women reach seventy years of age in one hospital market, the likelihood they have undergone a hysterectomy is 20 percent; while in another market it is 70 percent. In Iowa, the chances that male residents who reach age eighty-five have undergone prostatectomy range from a low of 15 percent to a high of more than 60 percent in different hospital markets. In Vermont, the probability that resident children will undergo a tonsillectomy has ranged from a low of 8 percent in one hospital market to a high of nearly 70 percent in another.

By contrast, the low-variation procedures derive from quite specific conditions for which there is a professional consensus on the preferred place or style of treatment. Prime examples are surgical repair of inguinal hernia and hospitalizations for hip fractures. For these conditions, practice style, at least in the United States, only plays a small part in affecting demand. As a general rule, diagnosis is not difficult. If the patient seeks medical care, variations in clinical judgments are constrained by a consensus. For inguinal hernia, the treatment is an operation. For hip fractures, virtually all patients are hospitalized.* The rates show little variation between hospital markets.

I developed the practice style theory after it became clear to me that the variation phenomenon could not be explained adequately by traditional theories. For example, consumer or population factors do not explain much of the difference in utilization rates among local hospital markets. Household interview studies in Vermont and Manitoba, Canada, compared the characteristics of residents living in high- and low-rate market areas. These studies failed to show correlations between service use rates and illness rates, insurance coverage, access to service, and other demand-related attributes of patients or populations. The variations also persist after adjustment for age, which tends to account for most illness-related differences in populations. While some variation in the use rate of specific procedures is explained by the per

---

*The specific treatments for hip fractures, however, show substantial variations. Choices of treatments include open or closed reduction (each can be done with or without internal fixation of the bone) and replacement of the hip joint with an artificial joint.

capita supply of facilities and physicians, most remains unexplained (5). For example, Noralou Roos has shown that the per capita number of beds and gynecologists are virtually the same in hospital markets with low and with high per capita hysterectomy rates (6).

The variation phenomenon appears to be worldwide, not explained by incentives associated with fee-for-service medicine. Even though obvious differences exist in the supply of surgeons, the organization and financing of services, and in the cultural and demographic characteristics of area residents, the pattern of variation for common procedures is similar among fee-for-service hospital markets in Iowa, Maine, Massachusetts, Rhode Island, and Vermont; among health maintenance organizations in the United States; and among the health care regions in Canada, England, and Norway. There is one common factor: physicians in each of these areas of the world read the same medical literature, participate in the same scientific traditions, and share similar scientific uncertainties concerning the value of specific procedures.

The most direct evidence for the importance of practice styles in influencing utilization rates comes from natural experiments in which practice styles change following the feedback of information to physicians on the rates in their own and neighboring market areas. Changes have been documented for hysterectomy rates in Saskatchewan, Canada, and Maine; for tonsillectomy rates in Vermont and Maine; and for lens extractions in Norway. The evidence indicates that the changes occurred primarily because physicians took actions to modify their clinical policies (7). In one example, a letter received from hospital officials in Maine speaks directly to the importance of admission policies in influencing the demand for services and documents the effect of feedback:

> We are following up after an ongoing one-year audit [of] hysterectomies [concerning] the high numbers of hysterectomies. [The past experience] in no way reflects the [current] actual numbers. The department of OB/GYN has set its own goals of between 220 and 240. This past year, 229 hysterectomies were completed during that period. Also, we have met our own criteria regarding the number of hysterectomies showing normal pathology at 20 percent to 25 percent. During this one-year period, a percentage of 24.9 was reached.

In the year prior to feedback, the market area served by this hospital had a rate of 118 procedures per 10,000 women, which was more than double the state average. In 1981, the year the letter discusses, the rate was 58, less than half the previous rate but 25 percent higher than the 1981 state average.

The value of the practice style theory is further illustrated by its power to provide a reasonable interpretation for the relative variation observed for rates of hospitalization. Clinicians will recognize an association between the order of the listing of causes of admission, ranked by the measure of variation in rate of admission, and the degree of discretion that physicians can exercise in the decision to hospitalize or not. At the lower end of the variation scale are admissions for hip fracture and for myocardial infarction. For these conditions, there is little choice; under current standards for care in the United States, patients must be hospitalized. But in the high range of variation—those causes of admission that are more variable than hysterectomy—the situation is not so clear-cut. For example, many cases of bronchitis, or of fracture of the forearm, can be and often are treated in the ambulatory setting; it is quite reasonable to infer that the range in variation for these causes of admission reflects differences in local practice styles. For the examples of causes of admission that rank at the extreme high end of the variation scale, the governing importance of professional decision making in determining the use rates of hospital resources speaks for itself.

Table 4.1 illustrates an important feature of the variation phenomenon: high-variation profiles are the rule, not the exception. When the "black box" is examined, most of the individual contents of medical practice—as defined by conventional classification systems—are more variable than hysterectomy. For example, when all medical, surgical, and pediatric hospitalizations are examined, less than 13 percent of cases are for causes that show less variation than hysterectomy; 12 percent are more variable than tonsillectomy. Most surgical as well as diagnostic procedures are also high variation. So much for the idea that most medical services are undifferentiated necessities, dispensed according to scientific norms.

To understand the cost implications of the practice style factor, let us return to the case of hysterectomy. Over the last decade, about 2,500 more hysterectomies were performed in one Maine market area, with about 35,000 women in the eligible age range, than would have been performed if the practice style of physicians located in a low-rate neighboring market had applied. At the current market value of approximately $4,000 per hysterectomy, this translates into a cost of $10 million. Yet the price of hysterectomy in this high-rate market is below average. Under DRG prospective pricing plans and preferred provider strategies, the hospitals in the high-rate market will be rewarded for their "efficiency." Yet the data show that the most important determinants of variations in per capita costs, or the "bottom line" for payers, are physicians' decisions to admit patients to the hospital or to employ a specific treatment, not the decisions they or other health care providers may make that affect the efficiency of medical care as reflected in the unit price of service or the length of a hospital stay.

TABLE 4.1. Medical and Surgical Causes of Admissions Ranked in Ascending Order of Variation in Incidence of Hospitalization (1980–1982)

Medical Causes of Admission	Surgical Causes of Admission
Low Variation	*Low Variation*
None	Inguinal and femoral hernia repair
	Hip repair except joint replacement
Moderate Variation	*Moderate Variation*
Acute myocardial infarction	Appendicitis with appendectomy
Gastrointestsinal hemorrhage	Major small and large bowel surgery
Specific cerebrovascular disorders	Gall bladder disease with cholecystectomy
	Adult hernia repairs except inguinal and femoral
High Variation	*High Variation*
Nutrional and metabolic diseases	Hysterectomy
Syncope and collapse	Major cardiovascular operations
Respiratory neoplasms	Pediatric hernia operations
Cellulitis	Hand operations except ganglion
Urinary tract stones	Foot operations
Cardiac arrhythmias	Lens operations
Miscellaneous injuries to extremities	Major joint operations
Angina pectoris	Stomach, esophageal, and duodenal operations
Toxic effects of drugs	Anal operations
Psychosis	Female reproductive system reconstructive operations
Heart failure and shock	Back and neck operations
Seizures and headaches	Soft tissue operations
Adult simple pneumonias	
Respiratory signs and symptoms	
Depressive neurosis	
Medical back problems	
Digestive malignancy	
G.I. obstruction	
Adult gastro-enteritis	
Peripheral vascular disorders	
Red blood cell disorders	
Adult diabetes	
Circulatory disorders exc. AMI, with card. cath.	

(*Continued*)

Since more than 85 percent of hospitalizations classified under the DRG system appear to have greater variation in per capita use rates among hospital market areas than hysterectomy, the above example is a conservative demonstration of the problems that attend unit pricing approaches to cost containment. Indeed, through the incentives they create for reducing lengths of stay in hospitals—thus freeing beds to allocate to new patients—cost-containment programs that focus only on the reduction of unit price may add to rather than reduce the overall costs. If hospitals that stand to lose money under the DRG system are able to improve their financial status by increasing the volume of ser-

TABLE 4.1. (Continued)

Medical Causes of Admission	Surgical Causes of Admission
Very High Variation	**Very High Variation**
Deep vein thrombophlebitis	Knee operations
Adult bronchitis and asthma	Transurethral operations
Organic mental syndromes	Uterus and andenexa operations
Chest pain	Extraocular operations
Transcient ischemic attacks	Misc. ear, nose, and throat operations
Kidney and urinary tract infections	Breast biopsy and local excision for nonmalignancy
Acute adjustment reaction	D & C, conization except for malignancy
Minor skin disorders	
Trauma to skin, subcut. tiss. and breast	
Chronic obstructive lung disease	T & A operations except for tonsillectomy
Hypertension	Tonsillectomy
Adult otitis media and URI	Female laparoscopic operations except for sterilization
Peptic ulcer	Dental extractions and restorations
Disorders of the biliary tract	Laparoscopic tubal interruptions
Pediatric gastroenteritis	Tubal interruption for nonmalignancy
Pediatric bronchitis and asthma	
Atherosclerosis	
Pediatric otitis media and URI	
Pediatric pneumonia	
Chemotheraphy	

Note: Cause of hospitalizations are taken from the diagnostic-related disease classification system, but cases have been grouped without regard to presence or absence of significant complication. Obstetrical and neonatal causes of hospitalization are excluded. Ranking is according to the systematic component of variation. Variations are measured across thirty hospital markets. The exhibit lists individually only those with more than 1,500 cases. More than 50 percent of hospitalizations are represented in the exhibit. Classes of variation are defined such that the variation associated with the first entry in a class is significantly more variable than the first entry in the previous class. For additional information, see K. McPherson, J. E. Wennberg, O.B. Hovind, and P. Clifford, *New England Journal of Medicine* 307 1310–14 (1982).

vices, then the inevitable result will be an acceleration in the rate of increase in per capita expenditures.

THE FIRST STEP:
MONITORING PERFORMANCE IN HOSPITAL MARKETS

Hospital markets are thus characterized by highly variable rates of use for most specific medical treatments, diagnostic tests, and surgical procedures, and by widely different resource use rates. The actions that are needed to reduce variation pertain to the clinical management and resource allocation decisions in specific hospital markets. The first step is to monitor and distribute information on the per capita performance in local hospital markets so that decision making can be modified when appropriate.

The essential features of the monitoring I propose are contained in health insurance records such as Medicare, Medicaid, and Blue Shield claims systems and hospital discharge abstracts similar to those used in the DRG program. Population counts and information on hospital resources, including annual budgets, numbers of facilities, and personnel also are needed. For outcome reports, information on survival must be joined to discharge data and to claims data to establish the link between use of medical care, diagnoses, and outcome. Sources for this information exist in many parts of the country and, for the Medicare program, nationwide.

The data should first be used to determine the geographic origin of patients who seek care at specific hospitals. The individual communities of a county or state are then arranged into hospital market areas such that most hospitalizations of local residents occur within area hospitals (and are thus initiated by physicians practicing within the area). Following this strategy, my colleagues and I have defined some two hundred hospital markets in the six New England states and over one hundred in the state of Iowa. The way the markets are organized assures a close association between the medical care experience of the local population and decisions made by health planners, regulators, local administrators, hospital trustees, clinicians, and, potentially, business coalitions. Since information on resource allocation and service use rates is available from all relevant places where care is given (whether in- or out-of-area), the per capita rates are truly population based and thus may be validly compared.

What do the reports look like? There are three kinds of reports. One series describes the status of resource allocations to specific communities: the number of hospitals, of hospital beds, expenditures, and hospital personnel, or the number of physicians invested, per capita, in the health care of the local communities. In reviewing the reports, it is important for the reader to understand that virtually all of the hospitalization experience of the resident population is accounted for even if it takes place at hospitals located in other areas. The reports can be used to project the per capita consequences of specific planning or regulatory decisions. They can also be used in cost-containment strategies to reduce expenditures in high-cost markets by cutting or stabilizing the local hospital industry as indicated by its contribution to the total numbers of personnel and beds per capita. Variations in these indicators are strongly correlated with per capita expenditures; with this information, hospital administrators and trustees can make a direct connection between plant size and employment complements in their specific hospitals and the variations in the total per capita costs.

The reports inevitably raise issues concerning the relationship between the quality of care and the level of resource investment, particularly if the comparisons are between markets with a high proportion of patients who are treated in a university teaching hospital. The New Haven market area, for example, ranks in the middle third of all market areas in Connecticut, largely because of its relatively low total numbers of beds and personnel per capita. Contrast this to the situation in Boston where the per capita expenditures are more than double: in New Haven, in 1978, the estimate was $215; in Boston it was $448. The beds allocated to the population of Boston number 4.5 per 1,000 while in New Haven they number only 2.7. The number of employees per 1,000 shows about a twofold variation.

The differences in resource use are not intuitively known by those on the scene. I have asked clinicians who have practiced in both Yale and Harvard teaching hospitals to estimate the per capita expenditures in each market. Their answers indicate they have no awareness of the magnitude of the difference; what is more surprising, many do not accurately guess which of the two markets is the more expensive. Nor can the difference be appreciated through the use of traditional indicators of performance, whose validity as measures of market consumption rates depends on the degree to which they correlate with the per capita market rates. Small-area research indicates their virtual independence. For example, among the hospital markets of a state, the occupancy rates of local hospitals, their average length of stay, and such measures of efficiency as the number of patients treated per bed (properly weighted to measure each hospital's relative contribution to the total experience) show little relationship with per capita number of beds or patient days, inpatient expenditures, and reimbursements per capita.

A second series of reports is concerned with the utilization of specific services for surgical and diagnostic procedures and for causes of admission. Table 4.2 gives an example for diagnostic procedures, showing the rate of use of cystoscopic examination among Medicare residents in twelve Maine markets defined for urology services (1976–77). The information is compiled from claims data from the Medicare Part B program and the Medicare enrollment file. Note that the cystoscopic rate in the Rumford market is more than double the rate for the state as a whole, while the Waterville rate is only about 54 percent of the average. The range of variation for the volume component (the per capita use rate, given here as the standardized procedure rate) varies by a factor of more than four, while the efficiency component—the average reimbursement per cystoscopy (not shown in table 4.2)—varies by less than 20 percent. This is typical of most surgical and diagnostic procedures and illustrates the importance of taking the volume into account in the design of cost-containment efforts. The information also

TABLE 4.2. Rates for Cystoscopies among Maine Medicare Enrollees by Urology Market Area of Residence, 1976–1977

Urology Market Area	Enrollees	Number of Exams	Rate	Ratio to State Average	% Enrollees with one or More Exams
Portland	43,192	1,641	3.8	1.33	2.8
Bangor	29,814	857	2.9	1.00	1.8
Lewiston	16,397	328	2.0	0.70	1.5
Augusta	9,920	235	2.4	0.83	1.7
Waterville	12,886	201	1.5	0.54	1.2
Biddeford	8,212	315	3.8	1.34	2.6
Rumford	3,895	232	5.9	2.08	3.9
Presque Isle	6,361	143	2.9	0.78	1.6
Skowhegan	4,203	95	2.3	0.79	1.6
Ellsworth	2,805	68	2.4	0.85	1.5
Caribou	5,757	125	2.2	0.76	1.8
Calais	1,969	23	1.2	0.41	1.0
State	156,325	4,478	2.86	1.00	2.0

raises questions concerning the effectiveness and efficacy of the various practice styles. Note that in Rumford, nearly 4 percent of enrollees had cystoscopic examinations, while in Waterville and Calais about 1 percent of enrollees were examined. What are the risks and benefits of these different patterns of use for this technology? We simply don't have a good answer to that question.

Similar tables have been generated from Medicaid and Blue Shield programs for use in feedback to Maine physicians. Under the feedback strategy I suggest, tables such as these should be generated by third-party carriers for all commonly used diagnostic and therapeutic procedures.

Hospital discharge data should also be used to generate age-adjusted utilization experiences for specific causes of admission or surgical procedures. Table 4.3 provides a sample report useful for feedback in a DRG-based prospective reimbursement program designed to draw attention to the importance of admission policies. Note that for medical back problems (DRG 243), the rate in the Portland and Lewiston hospital market areas is less than 60 percent of the average, while in the Augusta and Waterville area it is more than 30 percent higher than the average. Portland area residents experienced over 560 fewer cases than expected from the state average. The cost implications of the variations in admission rate for DRG-based reimbursement programs are also illustrated in this table. Over the two-year period, reimbursements for the Portland population under a DRG reimbursement program would be over $1 million less than expected from the state average. In Waterville and Augusta, their combined excess in reimbursements would be $500,000 more than expected. If the Portland use rate were the stan-

TABLE 4.3. Variations in Expected Admissions to Hospital for Selected Conditions in Nine Maine Hospital Markets, 1980–1981

Market Areas	Back Problems			Dental Extractions and Restorations		
	Admissions Observed −Expected[a]	Standard Rate	Reimburs. Observed −Expected (×$1,000)	Admission Observed −Expected[a]	Standard Rate	Reimburs. Observed −Expected (×1,000)
Portland	−567.1*	0.58	−1,048	−149.8*	0.49	−122
Bangor	−61.9	0.91	−108	−81.9*	0.48	−66
Lewiston	−283.9*	0.59	−503	−108.2*	0.29	−87
Augusta	+162.8*	1.32	+288	−42.0*	0.60	−33
Waterville	+150.6*	1.37	+267	−55.1*	0.43	−44
Biddeford	−74.0*	0.81	−131	+88.6*	2.10	+71
Brunswick	−10.3	0.96	−18	+115.9*	2.90	+93
Rockland	+2.7	1.01	+5	+60.0*	2.30	+48
Farmington	−74.0*	0.66	−131	−37.7*	0.24	−30
All Other	1,755.1*	1.27	+1,339	+172.1*	1.18	+140

Note: The input to the table is hospital discharge data, maintained by the Maine Health Information Center, and population data from the 1980 census. The nine markets examined are the most populated in the state. DRG-specific reimbursement rates are estimated using charge data from the Maryland Hospital Cost Commission for 1980. Column 2 gives the actual number of cases observed among residents of each market area subtracted from the expected number. A plus means more cases than expected, a minus, less. An asterisk indicates that the difference is statistically significant (p < .01). The expected number is the age-adjusted number of cases that would have occurred to area residents if the state rate had applied. The standardized utilization rate gives the age-adjusted rate for each area expressed as a ratio to the state average. Reimbursements above or below expected are estimated by multiplying the average charge for these DRGs for Maryland by the number of cases above or below expected.
[a] Observed minus expected, standardized to state average = 1.00
* Significant (p<.01)

dard, outlays for medical back admissions in Maine in 1980–81 would have been $7.7 million. If the Waterville rate were the standard, $18.2 million would have been expended. Such reports should be used in DRG programs to bring the variance to the attention of practicing physicians, hospital administrators, and other interested parties. The importance of admission rates in determining expenditures is clearly revealed here: more than 63 percent of the causes of hospitalization have admission rates that are more variable than medical back problems.

Dental extractions are among the most variable of causes of admission. Note in table 4.3 the more than tenfold range in variation in the standardized utilization rates among the nine individually listed markets. Per capita reimbursements under a DRG program would range from a low of $180 per 1,000 people to a high of $1,860. If the practice style in the Augusta area were the standard for the state, the costs in Maine for this service performed in the hospital setting would be about

$375,000; if the practice style for Brunswick were the standard, the reimbursements would be ten times higher, or about $3.7 million. Decreasing the use of hospitals for such high-variation procedures offers the potential for large reductions in the cost of hospital care. Reports such as these that identify points where savings can be realized should be used in cost-containment efforts.

A third series of reports is concerned with outcomes. As I have indicated, the practice style factor can play an important role in clinical decision making because the scientific evidence on the consequences of using particular treatments is ambiguous or incomplete. Estimates of survival and complication rates following the use of specific treatments for representative populations are frequently not available, even though they are essential for the evaluation of the common practices of medicine as well as for new technology. Claims data offer an inexpensive means for closing this information gap.

Claims data can be used, for example, for evaluating survival prospects or the probability of a secondary operation following the initial treatment of hypertrophy of the prostate by prostatectomy. I have used the Medicare claims data for such purposes in Maine, finding that the mortality rate in the year following prostatectomy was considered higher than predicted by most of the published literature. The probability of undergoing a second prostatectomy was also quite high, reaching 13 percent by the end of the fifth year. Such information can help physicians deal with the uncertainties revealed by the practice variation phenomenon, leading to a fuller understanding of the consequences of particular decisions and motivating physicians to take the necessary additional steps to improve the scientific basis of medical practice. Reports based on claims data for analysis of survival and complication rates should become routinely available for technology assessment and the evaluation of the consequences of the natural experiments that derive from variations in medical practice.

Is it possible to feed back information to physicians efficiently? Although this idea was first proposed by William Farr and Florence Nightingale well over one hundred years ago, recent advances in computer technology, biostatistics, and epidemiology only now make it feasible to produce routinely the reports I am recommending here. Furthermore, the necessary data are now becoming available in many parts of the country. Large, computerized, population-based data files, comprising hospital discharge records and health insurance claims, now exist in the public and private sectors. Several large states—California, Maryland, Massachusetts, New Jersey, New York, and Iowa—now have statutes that require hospitals to submit information on the cases they treat to publicly controlled data bases. Public use data bases have been key in our efforts to initiate feedback in the state of Maine.

American corporations, particularly large employers such as the American Telephone and Telegraph company, are beginning to employ their own records as a means for managing employee benefit packages. But for purposes of monitoring the activities of local markets, corporate data bases, used by themselves, have severe limitations because, as a rule, no single corporation has enough employees to allow for valid statistical inferences on practice variations in specific hospital markets. Rather, corporations and business or labor coalitions that want to use hospital market data in their cost-containment strategies should support the development of public data bases on a regional or statewide basis, as exemplified by the Maine Health Information Center. They could also promote information feedback by using their influence as large purchasers of care to insist that third-party carriers publish reports on expenditures and service use rates in local hospital markets.

Because of its national coverage and the richness of its data base, the Medicare program offers the best immediate opportunity to implement feedback in all parts of the country. The federal government now requires each hospital to record uniform information on the costs, reasons for hospitalization, and treatments for each hospitalization reimbursed under the Medicare program. When this information is linked to claims data under the Medicare Part B program and to patient registration files, a registry is created of the medical care events and certain outcomes for virtually the entire population of the United States who are sixty-five years and older. The many problems for public policy concerning the equity and outcome of care that are illustrated by the variation phenomenon, as well as the federal government's own need for effective cost containment, lead me to recommend that this very important national resource be used for this purpose.

THE SECOND STEP:
DEALING WITH THE EFFECTIVENESS PROBLEM

My plan for dealing with the effectiveness problem envisions the broad-based feedback of information on practice variations and outcomes targeted to state medical associations, specialty societies, and to individual hospitals and their physicians. My hypothesis is that this will result in the reconsideration of the indications for specific services. Some controversies concerning the need for or value of specific practices will be resolved through a critical review of the medical literature or by the application of decision analysis leading to the emergence of more objective standards. I expect that such standards, when applied within the context of a review of use rates in specific local markets, will result in a reduction in variation. For other services, reviews of the literature and the use of decision analysis will identify the controversies and the points of missing data, but they cannot, because of the lack of information, lead to a meaningful scientific consensus on the outcome implications. This process will, however, greatly refine the debate, identifying the critical uncertainties, and it should lead the profession to take the necessary steps to obtain more information.

Are these reasonable expectations? Can one expect that state medical societies, specialty organizations, practicing physicians, and academic medicine will pay attention and take action? I am confident that when information is presented in an objective fashion, physicians will respond by accepting responsibility for the outcome implications of the practice variation phenomenon. I have had occasion to bring specific information on hospital market areas to the attention of the state medical organizations in Vermont, Maine, and Iowa. In Iowa, this may be leading to an important cost-containment program based on provider initiative. In Vermont and Maine, it led to official action by the state medical organizations to endorse the routine feedback of information and to specific proposals to develop programs to deal with efficacy issues raised by the variations.

In the early 1970s, when Alan Gittelsohn and I first learned about the large variations in tonsillectomy rates in Vermont, I took the information to the elected officials of the Vermont Medical Society. Without formal program support, the society circulated the information on tonsillectomy rates to Vermont hospitals. As a result, two practicing physicians in Morrisville, Vermont, which was identified in the study as the high-rate area, undertook a review of the recent literature and concluded that indication standards for the procedure should be tightened. They convinced their colleagues that hospital policy on the use of tonsillectomy should be changed and that the procedure should be used only after a second opinion was obtained. In subsequent years, the rate for tonsillectomy dropped to less than 10 percent of the rate as first measured. This important example of physician-initiated response to information occurred without economic sanctions and was motivated primarily by concern that local practice patterns should conform to state-of-the-art criteria for recommending tonsillectomy.

When we first learned of the practice variations in Maine, we were invited by Daniel Hanley, who was then executive secretary of the Maine Medical Association and editor of the Maine Medical Journal, to write a series of articles setting out the variation phenomenon for Maine physicians. Hanley's initiative, first in publicizing the variations and then in organizing the physicians of Maine into a program to deal with the efficacy issues that variations raise, exemplifies the leadership that practicing physicians can provide. Financial support from the Commonwealth Fund made it possible to undertake a pilot project that initiated the systematic feedback of information and provided the opportunity to demonstrate that practicing physicians are willing to participate in the steps I outlined above to understand the outcome implications of variations. The success and popularity of the pilot project have convinced the Maine Medical Association that it should assume long-range responsibility for running the program of feedback and practice review.

The strategy is to bring together physicians from market areas with high and low rates for highly variable procedures to discuss the reports on practice variations. Focusing first on the published literature, can consensus be reached on the significance of the variations and a plan devised for reducing marginally indicated services? If the group concludes that an area is underserviced, how can the problem be corrected? If consensus cannot be reached, what additional information is required? Can information on survival and complication rates narrow the range of uncertainty? Are prospective studies needed to fill in the gaps? When uncertainties remain, can valid clinical trials be organized to resolve the question of efficacy?

The actions of the physicians convened to study variations in prostatectomy rates answer some of these questions. Although prostatectomy rates varied by a factor of more than 2.5 among hospital markets in Maine, consensus on the appropriate rate could not be reached through review of the literature. A basic uncertainty concerned the survival rate after surgery. Most reports suggest that the mortality rate attributable to this procedure is about 1.2 percent, but this estimate is based on in-hospital experience prior to discharge. A consensus emerged among these physicians that these patients were better treated by more conservative methods.

The physicians have also studied the evidence underlying their assumptions about the benefits of prostatectomy, particularly the expected gains in the patients' quality of life. Again finding gaps in the literature, they have been motivated to undertake a study to ascertain the objective as well as the subjective responses of their patients to the surgery. Currently being designed with the assistance of academic collaborators, this study will represent the first large-scale, population-based follow-up to document nonfatal outcomes associated with the use of this procedure. When completed, the study will help all physicians make better decisions about when to recommend prostatectomy as well as pinpoint remaining uncertainties that may need to be settled by a clinical trial.

The active involvement of Maine physicians in examining practice variations is indicative of the response to be expected from most medical practitioners. The special status of the medical professional derives partly from the exercise of collective responsibility for understanding illnesses and the consequences of alternative therapies, and for helping patients obtain the medical care they truly want. The professional uncertainties and disputes about outcomes that underlie some examples of variations present an intellectual challenge to practicing physicians as well as to researchers. They also indicate that past efforts to distinguish the scientific from the unscientific claims concerning effectiveness have not been sufficient; greater efforts are needed to base clinical choices on sound estimates of outcome probabilities and on values that correspond closely to patient preferences. My experiences indicate that information on practice variations, when used in a program of feedback that includes epidemiological, biostatistical, educational, and financial support, motivates practicing physicians to take the necessary steps to improve clinical decision making.

The uncertainties about clinical outcomes are particularly important for academic medicine because of its special responsibility for the science of medicine. If, as I propose, the feedback of information on service use variation is broadened to include the populations served primarily by prominent teaching institutions, interest in the significance of the variation phenomenon may be considerably enhanced. Intellectual curiosity and the need to justify differences in costs should lead naturally to sophisticated efforts to explicate the significance of the differences in practice styles.

There are other reasons why the variations should be of interest to academic medicine, not the least being their responsibility for the training of new physicians. In my opinion, the state of intellectual confusion on the rational use of medical services evidenced by the monitoring of local market performance calls upon academic medicine to increase the attention and support it gives to the disciplines involved in improving clinical decision making—to clinical epidemiology, biostatistics, and clinical decision analysis. An important topic for the research agenda is how to improve methods for evaluating health care outcomes, particularly means for measuring functional status. Today's dilemmas stem, in part, from advances in biomedical research. The natural next step is to improve the quality of research to examine the effect of these investments.

There are also implications for medical education. Medical students need more education in the methods of evaluating clinical decisions and their outcomes so they may assess for themselves the strengths and weaknesses of the various practice styles they will encounter in the course of their clinical training and prepare for their own contributions to resolving clinical uncertainties as practicing physicians.

Practicing physicians and their medical associations cannot act without broad-based support. Private philanthropy is playing a crucial role by providing leadership in mobilizing opinion on the importance of the practice variation problems. Examples include the Milbank Memorial Fund's investment in the development of clinical epidemiology; the support of the Commonwealth Fund, the Robert Wood Johnson Foundation, and the John A. Hartford Foundation to find solutions in basic research; as well as demonstration projects such as the Maine Medical Association project. With few other exceptions, however, there is currently little support in the private or public sector for the research needed to establish the outcome value of common medical practices.

The federal government's lack of effective policy is noteworthy. The National Center for Health Care Technology, whose agenda was technology assessment, has been abandoned, and funding for the National Center for Health Services Research, which has supported much of the research upon which my work is based, is minuscule in comparison to the need. The Health Care Financing Administration invests little or none of its research resources in projects concerned with the health outcome value of the services it pays for.

The failure of technology assessment to attract public support is all the more surprising in view of the implications of the uncertainty concerning surgical mortality. For example, if the conservative approach to prostatectomy observed in some New England areas were the national norm, the number of postoperative deaths in the United States would be about 1,900; with a more "aggressive" approach the number would be about 6,800, suggesting that under the high-rate strategy about 1 percent of American males over age sixty-five would die postoperatively. Most prostatectomies are paid for by the federal government. The public interest is served by a better understanding of the implications of the variations. The responsibility for furthering research into the outcome implications seems to rest in part with the federal government because many of its activities promote the public's use of health care.

THE THIRD STEP:
DEALING WITH THE COST-CONTAINMENT PROBLEM

Many hospitalized patients can be effectively and safely treated in the ambulatory setting; the problem is knowing who they are. The shift of such patients to the ambulatory setting will neither disrupt the patient-physician relationship nor have a significant negative economic impact on physicians. Given the current imperatives to contain the costs of medical care and reallocate resources to more productive ends, it should be in most peoples' interest to reduce the use of hospitals for marginally indicated causes of admission and to translate the reduction in demand into stabilization of hospital per capita costs by appropriately controlling the capacity of hospital markets. This can occur only with the active cooperation of the medical profession.

Government officials, managers of benefit plans, and representatives of public or private interest groups can exercise influence in persuading the medical profession of the need to respond to the challenge. But lacking a detailed understanding of the nature of medical choices, they are in no position to deal with such specific issues as the necessity for hospitalization in a specific hospital market. Given information on practice patterns in their local and regional hospital markets, a broad consensus may emerge that it is both safe and in the public interest to reduce the hospitalization rate for many high-variation causes of admission.

This hypothesis needs to be tested. The feedback reports give the information necessary for action; they identify the hospital markets with costly practice styles for specific discretionary admissions, and they identify hospital markets with costly administrative practices with regard to hospital expenditure, bed, and personnel rates.

There are concurrent options for the private sector to help control the capacity of local hospital markets and to motivate providers to pay attention to high-variation causes of hospitalization. Perhaps the single most important step is to ensure the feedback of information itself. As I have mentioned, business and labor coalitions are well situated to play a role in organizing the necessary pressure. And when adequate information is available, as in Iowa, such groups offer an important focus for the educational efforts needed to translate the information into action by community leaders, whether they are representatives of individual firms, hospital trustees, or members of planning or regulatory commissions.

In some circumstances, corporations may possess the necessary strength to bring about change virtually on their own. In Maine, a number of smaller hospital markets have consistently elevated per capita expenditure, personnel, and bed rates. In several of these markets, pulp and paper companies employ a large percentage of local residents. Interest is growing on the part of these companies to reduce health benefit expenditures (in part because decentralization of the actuarial base of employee benefits has meant that health care benefit outlays are now allocated against local plant budgets, making the differences in per

capita expenditures a matter of greater concern to local managers) (8).*
Hospital discharge reports from the Maine Health Information Center are being used by at least one paper company to plan strategies for reducing corporate costs. It will be interesting to see whether these efforts will shift costs to employees or to other local residents or result in direct pressures on the local hospital industry to control its capacity, thus controlling costs for all members of the community. The influence of these corporations includes substantial representation on hospital boards of trustees, so they are in a position to promote the rational cost-containment model proposed for Iowa. Together with labor leaders, these companies could also help create a wider constituency for effective cost containment by informing employees about the variation phenomenon, making them aware that some of their benefit dollars are used to purchase services that, if they lived in low-cost hospital markets, might be available for other purposes, such as an increase in take-home pay or other fringe benefits.

Government can also help bring pressure to bear. State governments can directly promote attention to the variation phenomenon by using their Medicaid management information system to create reports, by passing legislation to establish public data systems, and by using population-based reports in certificate-of-need programs and hospital rate-setting programs. The federal government can make some very important contributions to the needed reforms, in part by employing population-based utilization review by professional review organizations as mandated by law (P.L. 97-248). The use of DRG-specific feedback reports in this program would, in my opinion, effectively promote physician interest in the variation phenomenon and make providers as well as policymakers more sensitive to the importance of physician practice style in influencing the per capita reimbursement rates for most causes of hospitalization. These reports can be generated with very little cost to the government, using existing Medicare data.

SUMMARY

Most treatments, diagnostic tests, and surgical operations have highly variable use rates among hospital markets. One reason for the variation is professional controversy, disagreement on treatments that arises

---

*The rating of health insurance to reflect local market expenditure rates offers an opportunity to increase awareness of local planning and management decisions and serves to reduce transfer payments between market areas, thus promoting geographic equity. I have discussed these issues in detail elsewhere (8).

from ambiguous or incomplete scientific evidence on the value of specific services. To resolve such controversies—and to improve the opportunity for informed judgment on specific treatments—better information on the outcome of care is needed. A second reason for the variation phenomenon is the individualistic approach adopted by physicians for reasons of their own or their patient's convenience or because of their interpretation of the requirements for "defensive" medicine. The reduction in demand for hospitalization based on these reasons offers opportunities for large savings without fear that needed services are being withheld.

I have proposed a plan for dealing with the practice variation phenomenon based on the distribution of reports detailing per capita use rates for individual hospital market areas. The reports are population based, taking into account the total experience of the resident population—whether services are obtained locally or at out-of-area sources. The reports thus allow valid comparison between hospital markets in their hospitalization rates, including expenditure, bed, personnel, and service use rates for cases classified by DRGs or by surgical or diagnostic procedures. Experience with the use of such information in Maine and Vermont indicates that physicians become motivated to undertake serious reexaminations of the scientific basis for their clinical decisions and take actions to obtain more information on the outcome implications of common treatments. Such efforts by academic as well as practicing physicians hold promise for improving the scientific basis of medical practice.

Experience in Iowa suggests the feasibility of using the population-based reports as a means for identifying costly examples of the use of hospitals for marginal services that many physicians feel can be treated in the ambulatory setting or not at all. Particularly in high-use rate markets, a relatively large proportion of inpatient care is of this nature. If demand for these services can be reduced and the overall size of the local hospital industry stabilized, substantial savings would ensue. This requires the cooperation and initiative of the medical profession, who must make the highly selective choices concerning which cases do not require hospitalization. To be successful, hospital management and boards of trustees must respond with cost-saving administrative decisions. The plan will require broad-based support from patients' community leaders, business and labor groups, and government. Briefly, I have suggested the major element of that support should include the establishment of a system for the feedback of information, support for technology assessment efforts, and in the case of cost containment, active promotion of the effort to reduce the use of hospitals.

REFERENCES

1. Wennberg, J.E., Gittelsohn, A.M., and Shapiro, N. Health care delivery in Maine. 3: Evaluating the level of hospital performance. *J Maine Med Assoc* 66:298–306 (1975).
2. Wennberg, J.E., and Kimm, S. Common uses of hospitals: A look at Vermont. *In:* Harvard Child Health Project, *Children's Medical Care Needs and Treatments.* Cambridge, Mass.: Ballinger (1977).
3. McCracken, S., Latessa, P., and Wennberg, J.E. *A Study of Hospital Utilization in Iowa in 1980.* Des Moines: Shervi-Share of Iowa (1982).
4. Wilson, P., and Tedeschi, P. *Community Correlates of Hospital Use.* Health Services Research (in press).
5. McPherson, K., Strong, P.M., Epstein, A., and Jones, L. Regional variations in the use of common surgical procedures within and between England and Wales, Canada, and the United States. *Soc Sci and Med* 15A:273–88 (1981).
6. Roos, N.P. Hysterectomy: Variation in rates across small areas and across physicians' practices. *Am J Pub Hlth* 74:327–35 (1984).
7. Wennberg, J.E., Blowers, L., Parker, R., and Gittelsohn, A.M. Changes in tonsillectomy rates associated with feedback and review. *Pediatrics* 59:821–26 (1977).
8. Wennberg, J.E. Should the cost of insurance reflect the cost of use in local hospital markets? *New Eng J Med* 307:1374–81 (1982).

5 The Evaluation of Surgical Care

Francis D. Moore, M.D.

This chapter focuses on the assessment of the quality of surgical care. Despite its many imponderables, there are several important indices of quality available, some of which are adaptable to large regional or statewide data bases. It is no longer justified to consider quality assessment as beyond the reach of the inquisitive clinician or policy scholar in analyzing aggregates of patients or procedures. In any evaluation of clinical care, be it a special area such as cardiology, neurology, cardiac surgery, or neurosurgery or a more general field, the collaboration of clinicians experienced in the work and in its statistical base is essential for analysis and interpretation. Hospitals and staff groups whose work is logged in the data base should be informed of results and comparative judgments before general publication so that they may check out the adequacy of the data and be aware of their own departures from regional norms. Work in this area should not be thought of as surveillance or as a source of journal articles and scare headlines, but rather as a collaboration between regional data analysis, on the one hand, and the clinicians who are working at the public interface and responding to the complaints and needs of their patients, on the other.

In this chapter I will be principally concerned with access to health care as indicated by treatment frequencies corrected for patient demand, with data on the comparative use of operations in hospitals (where surgical operations are performed) rather than comparison among populations, with the analysis of the use of several approaches as opposed to a single treatment option for a disease complex, and with trend analysis over time. Outcomes and costs can be realistically interpreted when based on the clinical analysis of treatments undertaken.

Concepts discussed here have been sharpened during work performed at the Massachusetts Health Data Consortium with the assistance of the Walnut Medical Charitable Trust, the Jessie B. Cox Foundation, and the Robert Wood Johnson Foundation.

For reasons of space, discussion of these latter aspects (outcomes and costs) will necessarily be brief.

FREQUENCIES OF TREATMENT

Considered as a single variable, the frequency with which a treatment (such as the use of a drug or a surgical operation) is employed in a population is, in my opinion, meaningless. It certainly does not represent "practice style." Even if such a frequency ("rate") is compared with other similar areas, it is essentially meaningless if the epidemiology of disease in those small areas and the highly variable complaints arising therefrom (the demand factors) are not taken into consideration. But suitably couched in demand-factored ratios localized to hospitals and analyzed over time with all options considered, the patterns of physician response to patient demand become an index of the variable access to and supply of services. This is an important area of health research that should be undertaken only by the use of a method embodying both scientific and clinical sophistication. It carries an important and sometimes severe message for hospitals, physicians, third-party entrepreneurs, patients, and the public.

THE SMALL-AREA VARIATION METHOD

To Wennberg and colleagues must go full credit for publishing a very large number of papers on the method of small-area variation (SAV), essentially unmodified since its first use in 1971–72 and its adaptation from the earlier work of Lewis, published in 1969 (1–2). In my opinion, from the time of the first Wennberg-Gittelsohn publication in *Science* in 1973 (1), it has been clear that this method, although now widely used and reported in a large number of research papers, is flawed. The method examines the supply of a clinical service (usually a single surgical procedure) without regard to the demand for that service as indicated either by the epidemiology of the disease being treated or of complaints related thereto, and without regard to the use of alternative treatment options, the work of hospitals, annual variation, or outcomes. The method makes the tacit assumptions (never examined in any of the SAV papers) that all of the demand factors in American medicine are constant and that all variability is due to the "practice style" of physicians (3–5). In point of fact, neither assumption is valid.

The SAV method has avoided any data on the many other causes of variation. It has not localized the performance of operations to specific hospitals, evidently preferring to relate treatment rates to a regional, population, or "area" denominator. The SAV method reports the frequency of only one of several alternative treatment options for a given disease or complaint complex (usually this has been a surgical operation), neglecting all others, whether medical, surgical, further diagnosis, or temporizing. The SAV method usually has reported data for only one year (or for several months extrapolated to a year), overlooking important trend analysis and annual variability.*

In the limited scope available here, a brief critique of this method will be presented, including illustrative examples. This is essential as a preliminary to a description of an alternative method of treatment frequency analysis, called "treatment options and practice profiles." The major problems that I see with the SAV method will be discussed under several headings. Were all these "faults" to be rectified, there would assuredly still be variations in treatment frequency, but they would not be perceived as artifacts of the method or universally assigned to "practice style" (5).

Epidemiologic Constancy

The SAV method examines the supply of a treatment without regard to demand for treatment as based on the epidemiology of the disease to be treated. Western medicine has operated in a complaint-response mode for centuries. Complaints are engendered by disease and treatments are a response to such complaints that bring the patient to the physician. We cannot assume that this epidemiology is constant.

Examples. Carcinoma of the breast is commoner among upper-class white women of Northern European extraction than it is among Southern Europeans, African blacks, or Asiatics; fibroids of the uterus are commoner among black women than among white; hypertension is commoner among black men, but surprisingly, coronary artery disease is not; athletic injuries are much commoner in small areas where there are colleges and other educational institutions involving athletic programs; hearing defects are often localized to small areas; there have been areas where congenital disease such as extrophy of the bladder or Tetralogy of Fallot is remarkably frequent, presumably owing to in-

---

*The authors of the SAV literature have now made available the software of this method for the use of others, by sale or rental, through Codman Enterprises, Concord, New Hampshire. A complete SAV bibliography is not presented here for reasons of space; the references to this chapter include reviews and opinions (5), a small representative set of SAV literature (5–10), critiques and comments (3, 10–12) and some comments of Wennberg and his group in defense of the method (4, 13–15).

breeding over several generations; gallstones are much commoner in certain Indian tribes than in other groups. Lyme disease is commoner where there is an animal reservoir and a certain species of tick (locally highly variable), while cholera and typhus are commoner in seaports (towns or "areas" only a few miles away will be almost free of those diseases). These are but a tiny sampling of the thousands of examples of local disease variability that will bias treatment frequencies. Space does not permit a complete tabulation (with references) of all local epidemiologic variability in the United States. The assumption of disease constancy is one of the weakest aspects of the SAV method.

Frequency of Complaint

The SAV method makes no allowance for variability in the frequency of complaints. Even were the distribution of diseases constant in all small areas and communities—never proven and rarely the case—the distribution or frequency of complaints bringing patients to the physician is highly variable. Insofar as the SAV method interprets all variability as due to the "practice style" of physicians, it is clearly in error: identical physician response to variable complaint frequencies would produce variable treatment frequencies despite constancy of "practice style."

Examples. Angina pectoris is a complaint of a certain type of precordial pain often but not always related to demonstrable underlying occlusive coronary artery disease. Even though coronary artery disease might have a uniform population distribution throughout western countries—this is unproven—the distribution of angina pectoris shows a definite educational bias (16). Young executives in highly organized companies are warned by the company physician to consult a physician if they have the faintest twinge of precordial pain radiating down the arm or to the jaw. Populations of comparable age and sex who do outdoor work (for example, laborers, farmers, or fishermen) and who may less frequently be college graduates do not express this complaint as often. Since angina pectoris (along with other symptoms in a constellation of complaints) is the commonest indication for coronary bypass surgery, it is evident that the frequency of bypass operations may be determined in part by these factors that bias the complaint frequency of angina pectoris even in adjacent "small areas."

The same is true of minor vaginal bleeding of benign origin at the time of the menopause. Since this is often an indication either for hysterectomy or hormone therapy, it is important to inquire as to whether women around the time of the menopause will always come to the doctor with exactly the same degree of bleeding. As any gynecologist knows, there are differences in the sense of personal hygiene that brings women to the physician with irregular menses or vaginal bleeding. Like angina pectoris (though possibly not quite as clear-cut), early and prompt complaints of small amounts of vaginal "spotting" on the underclothes are characteristic of a more highly educated and in some cases a more affluent group. Other groups of women, sometimes in less fortunate circumstances and perhaps less fastidious, less prone to physician visits for minor symptoms, will await much more severe bleeding. The frequency of treatment including hysterectomy will vary accordingly.

A classic example of procedures whose frequencies are wholly determined by demand are tubal sterilization and vasectomy for sterilization. Here the patient comes to the physician asking for the treatment (i.e., sterilization). There is no "disease" being treated. The SAV authors have noted the great variability in this entity with some degree of wonder (17). One would naturally expect the request for sterilization to be somewhat lower in a devout Catholic community than in a neighboring Protestant or Jewish community. Here is a perfect example of the futility of reporting procedure variability without regard to demand, population differences, or, in this case, ethnic background and religion. Vasectomy and tubal sterilization are pure demand-generated procedures; there is no basis for variation in their distribution/frequency/epidemiology other than variation in patient demand.

Comparability of Populations

The SAV method assumes that all populations are comparable. Not only does this method neglect the epidemiology of disease and complaints resulting therefrom, but it also fails to take into consideration population characteristics such as educational status, affluence, occupation— white-collar versus blue-collar versus open-air labor (including sun exposure)—or housing.

Examples. The SAV authors have reported, for example, substantial differences in resource utilization for the hospital care of patients in Boston as compared with New Haven (14). Their statistical work consisted simply of a ratio of total population to total hospital budgets. It completely neglected the fact that New Haven is a community of about 143,000 (137,999 in 1970) people in which 12,000 to 14,000 (around 10 percent) are enrolled in the Yale University Health Plan (YHP). The city of New Haven has long had a tradition of admitting its Yale students to full voting rights and municipal participation. So the student population as well as the resident faculty appear in the population statistics. The Yale Health Plan is an effective HMO dealing with low-risk enrollees, many of them young healthy college students or young vigorous faculty. Many preventive medical steps are taken, and there is extensive use of ambulatory facilities. In addition, and possibly most important, many college students, if they are confronted with a serious illness or operation of the type that might demand extensive resource utilization, return to their home city for care by physicians familiar to their families.

By contrast, Boston has a population of about 700,000 (641,000 in 1970). To display a population mix comparable to New Haven, Boston would require 80,000 students covered by an HMO to live and vote in the city. This is not the case. Most of the students at Harvard and MIT live in Cambridge. Many of the students at Boston University and Tufts live in Brookline or other suburbs. At the time of the SAV study, there was no single or unified HMO involved with any large segment of the latter group of Boston students.

It is therefore hardly surprising that comparisons between these two different communities of different size, different economic and non-resident (student) makeup, and different referral patterns as well as different ethnic composition, show widely different utilization rates and costs per case.

Degree of Constancy

The SAV method reports variability of procedures without defining what degree of constancy is to be expected. It is assumed that variability is bad and constancy is good. What is the expectation of constancy in a treatment frequency when there are many variables and other treatment options? When treatments are undergoing change? What is the evidence to support the claim that frequencies should be expected to be constant, as between small population groups? What is the basis for a moral or quality judgment that variability is undesirable? In several instances where treatment options are very limited (femoral fracture, inguinal herniorraphy), there is little variation. Are we to expect that changing therapies should be exhibited at that degree of constancy (e.g., studies undertaken during the abandonment of radical mastectomy or of tonsillectomy)? Such changes (abandonment of old procedures and adoption of new ones) are initiated in teaching centers. Their effects are often delayed in smaller communities where the surgeons have been trained many years before. Where treatment mores are under change, a "ripple effect" will produce variability between small areas in and of itself. To somehow regulate treatment patterns to constancy as the SAV authors propose (18) would freeze the variance essential to the evolution of medicine.

Available Treatment Options

The SAV method overlooks the effect on variability of the number of treatment options available. In one such study reported from Massachusetts, the number of options available when plotted against observed variability made an almost linear series (19). The SAV studies have focused entirely on one procedure in each disease category, neglecting completely the use of its alternatives.

Examples. The treatment of vaginal bleeding of benign origin at the menopause involves choices among sixteen or eighteen different treatment options with or without operative procedures such as dilation and curettage (D&C) or hysterectomy. Each case is different; there can be no "consensus" among such a variety of complaints, diseases, and treatments. The SAV method reports only one frequency (hysterectomy). By contrast, fractures of the femur are always repaired by reduction and fixation so the patient can be mobilized. Immobilizing the patient, in bed, in traction, was abandoned about 1935. There is only one treatment option. The SAV authors have regarded this sort of constancy as evidence of "consensus." This is a misleading term in cases such as fracture of the femur or inguinal herniorrhaphy where but a single option is available. "Consensus" might be applied to such a thing as the choice of insulin preparations in juvenile diabetics or the election of digitalis derivatives in heart failure. When the SAV method undertakes the study of medicinal (i.e., medical versus surgical) treatment where a large number of options are available, much greater variability can be expected.

Annual Variation

The SAV reports are confined to a single year (or several months) in most journal articles, neglecting annual variation. In countering this criticism, SAV authors have employed a chart showing constancy of regional frequency in certain areas, overlooking completely those that demonstrate inconstancy over time (13–14).

Examples. A certain small community hospital in a Maine country town is the only hospital in its "small area." I have analyzed its record over the past twenty years for hemorrhoidectomy, herniorrhaphy, and cholecystectomy, among other procedures. It is interesting that in three operations this hospital varied in large swings of volume from year to year. Following SAV methods, with respect to hemorrhoidectomy, its area would have been the lowest in the state some years and the highest in the state in other years. Talking with the surgeons there, it is evident that their indications for hemorrhoidectomy are quite well considered and carefully executed, carrying out hemorrhoidectomy only in the more severe cases. The number of such severe cases coming in any one year is highly variable. Practitioners have long noted that complaint frequencies often tend to "run in groups."

Where annual variation is larger than the variation between areas, small-area variation data become meaningless. In much of the SAV literature, the data are in single numbers, or less than twenty procedures in a year. However, no amount of statistical sophistication can iron out the annual change in demand of a small number of patients, making it appear as a significant "small-area" aberration of "practice style."

Hospital-Specific Data

Relating data on treatment frequencies to population groups or "areas" rather than to hospitals tends to cover up important aberrancies of specific hospitals. This is the "band-aid" effect of SAV studies, covering up the very abnormalities that are most worrisome.

Examples. In an SAV study of surgical utilization in Massachusetts, one area was rated as normal (and at the state norm) for hysterectomy frequency (19). Further research disclosed that within this area, one hospital carries out hysterectomies on almost 46 percent of its total gynecologic discharges, whereas most of the other hospitals are between 15 and 22 percent. It is evident that the SAV method, in concentrating on "areas" and overlooking the work of specific hospitals, has missed an aberrancy that may have a significant health policy message. Even were this the only failing of the SAV method, it would argue strongly against its continued use. How many other normal "small areas" hide severely aberrant hospital practices within them? After an SAV study is completed, at great expense, the entire procedure must be repeated on a hospital basis if corrective steps are to be taken.

Epidemiologic Control

The SAV data associate treatment frequency variability with late survivorship, without adequate epidemiologic control.

Examples. In a Wennberg-Gittelsohn article in *Scientific American* on the late survival of patients having prostatectomy, it was claimed that postoperative patients have a higher late death rate than a life table-controlled normal population of males of the same age (20). This is hardly surprising, because prostatectomy cannot reverse the bladder changes, ureterovesical reflux, and ascending pyelonephritis that takes its toll in bladder neck obstruction due to prostatic hypertrophy. Yet the SAV authors interpret this as being a late mortality due to the treatment itself. The control group for this study should have been a group of men with high-grade prostatic obstruction who were not operated upon.

Standardization of Treatment Frequencies

The SAV method has claimed social and economic benefits from standardizing treatment frequencies at the lowest level in order to save money. But this conclusion does not take into account the fact that the low rates are frequently in underserved areas. In addition, "area" rates are themselves invalid because medicine is practiced by the physicians of the hospital staffs seeing individual patients *seriatum*, not treating large groups *en masse*. There is therefore no means to regulate treatment frequencies to the lowest level, even if this were felt to be desirable. The implication that money can be saved by withholding treatment was especially noticeable in the early SAV literature; now the authors ask, "Which rate is right?" (21). There is no way to answer this rhetorical question, as they provide no data on alternative treatments, on rehabilitation, or on clinical outcomes of treatment (early or late).

Examples. It has been shown that hip replacement is especially infrequent among poor rural blacks in Alabama. To maintain that all populations of the United States should have this operation carried out at that low frequency—conforming to the "most economical practice" but leaving them with severely symptomatic hips, painful in any position and inhibiting their normal activity as they grow older—is poor health policy in my opinion.

Policy Decisions

The SAV method leads to unwise policy decisions; its "feedback effect" has been overrated. As mentioned above, physicians see individual patients in sequence; they cannot relate the needs of one patient to treatment of a prior patient or to the several they will see next week. This is a fallacy of the "area" or population denominator, intrinsic to the SAV method. SAV authors claim that feedback of their information has resulted in a decline of various procedures (5). In many such cases, they have taken credit for declines due to entirely different factors. For example, the decline in tonsillectomy in Maine began in 1947 and has continued unabated for forty years (22). One cannot see in this curve any clear impact from the SAV publications.

THE METHOD OF TREATMENT OPTIONS AND PRACTICE PROFILES

As suggested at the outset, analysis of treatment frequencies should provide insight into access to and utilization of services and the possible exploitation of patients. Because its message is both important and potentially critical, reflecting on the reputations of hospitals or physicians, such analysis must be done with care and clinical sophistication. The method offered here is that of treatment options and practice profiles (TOPPS).

TOPPS is only one of several alternative methods that might be used in an analysis of treatment frequencies. These include direct physical examination and interviewing of large populations to determine what their needs are, the relation of treatments to expressed demands as indicated by patient visits, and finally patient treatment and outcomes. In other studies, the "idealized" uses of treatment (drugs, operations) have been defined by consensus panels and then compared with actual practices in various parts of the country. Neither of these methods (personal examination or "ideal" consensus) is adaptable to statewide computer-stored medical data bases.

The method of treatment options and practice profiles is a way of assessing treatment frequencies in surgery and possibly in other fields as well; my experience thus far has been entirely based on hospital discharge data for surgery and certain diagnostic interventions such as angiography. The TOPPS method depends first upon the selection of the candidate cohort (the denominator, persons most "at risk"), the evaluation of the use of several treatment options in that cohort, and the expression of two ratios that indicate the practice pattern. One is the ratio of treatments undertaken to suitable candidates coming to the physicians. The second ratio expresses the relative use of each treatment option. While TOPPS data are localized to hospitals in the first instance, "area" data can be derived once the hospital migration patterns for each area are known. The candidate cohort, expressed as a fraction of the population, gives the complaint frequency for a community whether large or small. It is itself a remarkably interesting index of the demand density for medical care. Since the data are localized to hospitals, it is possible to communicate directly with the hospitals exhibiting aberrant or asymmetrical clinical behavior (even though they are in "normal" areas) and to seek an understanding of practice patterns before publication or public criticism. The TOPPS method is always concerned with a series of successive years, avoiding the error of focusing on a few months or a single year. Various components of this method will be discussed briefly, including problems and difficulties identified as we establish the specific TOPPS ratio for initial studies.

Procedure for TOPPS Analysis

The Candidate Cohort

Definition. A candidate cohort is a group of patients admitted to a hospital or hospitals with a complaint/disease/diagnostic complex that defines them as potentially treatable by the treatment options under consideration. This is the population "at risk" for the procedure(s). It is a measure of the "demand" factor. The size of this candidate cohort in relation to the population of a region or area is the complaint frequency. This is a remarkably interesting datum in that it provides a first estimate of the distribution of demand densities bringing patients to physicians; in the case of individual hospitals, it gives an idea of their "case loading" in a particular specialty, diagnostic group, or symptom complex. The candidate cohort is the denominator of the treatment frequency ratio; it is therefore the demand factor in the treatment frequency ratio expressing the necessary background for the supply factor in the numerator. Its definition and its comparative analysis by aggregating various ICDA-9 or DRG clusters is central to the intelligent use of the TOPPS method in large statewide or regional data bases, including large numbers of community and hospital data subsets.

My experience has been with hospital discharge data only. This is clearly a limitation because a candidate cohort should ideally be based on the total number of patients with a particular complaint seeking physician visits and ambulatory care.

Examples. In *carcinoma of the breast,* the ideal candidate cohort would be all those patients coming to the physician or to the hospital with a complaint of a lump in the breast. Since the majority of breast lumps are found by the patient herself, this is a realistic complaint that is both a symptom and a sign. While there is no simple discharge coding proxy for such a broad group, treatment cannot be undertaken without a diagnosis based on breast biopsy. Therefore the total group of patients having breast biopsy (BBx) constitutes a valid proxy for the candidate cohort in treatment of breast disorder of any type. The fraction of biopsies positive for cancer (CaBx), is an important index in any diagnostic procedure. In the case of breast biopsy, rates of positivity over 30–35 percent have been considered as indicating that too few biopsies are being undertaken, while positivity rates below 7–10 percent have suggested that too many biopsies are being done. In any event, the use of the several treatment options for breast cancer (see below) can be expressed in relation to this basic candidate cohort of patients showing positive biopsies.

In the case of a candidate cohort for *hysterectomy,* our initial studies have employed the total gynecologic discharges (TGD) as a proxy for women coming with complaints in the set of symptom complexes and disease entities potentially treated by hysterectomy. This denominator can be refined further by subtracting from the total gynecologic discharges the women having dilation and curettage for pregnancy termination (DCA) and certain other specific subgroups (Bartholin's cyst, leukoplakia) of minor gynecologic procedures (MING). This type of refinement (i.e., narrowing definition) of candidate cohorts in each treatment cluster can only be established on the basis of experience with the data base at hand, and with expert clinical collaboration.

For *cesarean section,* the candidate cohort is obviously the total number of women in the third trimester of pregnancy, read out as the total birth rate—total live births (TLB) and its subset total pelvic deliveries (TPD)—in the area or the hospital. It is from this group that the obstetrician selects those women or fetuses that appear to mandate cesarean section. To relate cesarean section to gross populations without specifying the presence or absence of pregnancy is clearly fallacious. Age, religion, multiparity, and prior cesarean section will vary among small-area populations; the cesarean fraction of total deliveries must always be evaluated on the background of these and other clinical variables.

For *prostatectomy* the candidate cohort would ideally be all men who seek help because of dysuria (trouble voiding), suggesting bladder neck obstruction, with such symptoms as frequency, nocturia, dribbling, and incontinence. Again, such a broad data base would require access to physician office records. Despite this limitation, the cluster of discharge diagnoses of prostatic hypertrophy (PH), bladder neck obstruction (BNO), and obstructive uropathy (OU) does provide a candidate cohort; only some of these cases require open prostatectomy (OP) or transurethral prostatectomy (TUR), whereas others are treated with indwelling catheters (IDC) or antibiotics (AA).

In the case of chronic active (i.e., symptomatic) *coronary artery disease* (CAD), the development of the candidate cohort (excluding acute myocardial infarction) has involved six major components of discharge indexing as the principal ICDA-9-CM diagnoses. These "primary six" codes (CHD 6) are

1. angina pectoris (AP)
2. coronary atherosclerosis (CAS)
3. chronic coronary insufficiency (CCI)
4. unspecified chronic ichemic heart disease (CID)
5. intermediate coronary syndrome (ICS)
6. old myocardial infarction (OMI)

These six (when listed as a principal diagnosis) are the primary indices in the ICDA-9 system for chronic active coronary disease excluding acute myocardial infarction (AMI).

In addition, there is a secondary subset of five discharge diagnoses (SEC 5) that are potentially related to coronary disease (when indexed as the principal diagnosis). They are included only if one of the foregoing "primary six" are present as "markers" in the remaining subset of listed diagnoses for each case. These five additional diagnoses (three of which require "marker" identification) in the candidate cohort are

1. chest pain (plus "marker") (CP)
2. dysrythmia (plus "marker") (DYS)
3. heart failure (plus "marker") (CHF)
4. coronary procedure: bypass (BP) or angioplasty (APL) (with or without "marker" but with an unrelated principal diagnosis)
5. bypass or angioplasty as principal procedure but with no "marker" (i.e., coding error)

By programming these ICDA-9 codes in a statewide data base, it is possible to embrace all patients who are discharged from hospitals with chronic active coronary heart disease as their chief complaint or principal diagnosis. Overlap is avoided by basing selection on a single coronary identifier for each patient record in a hierarchical model; no record is counted twice. An additional inactive group has coronary heart disease as a historical or incidental finding, and a third group is admitted for acute myocardial infarction. None of these is included in the candidate cohort for elective bypass or angioplasty.

The choice of a candidate cohort and the selection of a suitable complex of codings, as well as some record-room research, are required before undertaking a study of this type. Currently, I am examining candidate cohorts for several other disease complexes. In each one the candidate cohort is designed to be computer identifiable from hospital discharges in large data bases and avoids overlap. Most large data bases are discharge specific rather than patient specific. Patients having more than one discharge in one year will count in the data as two or more units; suitable correction for this source of error can be made by random record-room sampling of each cohort to establish its rate of multiple discharges.

Treatment Options

Ideally, all of the treatment options available to the physician in dealing with a disease/complaint/diagnostic complex should be listed and analyzed for comparative use rates by hospitals and in regions. In most cases, this is impossible because of the lack of data on ambulatory care or medical treatments (e.g., drugs) that are not included in discharge-diagnosis coding systems. Even in "surgical" diseases such as hemorrhoids, treatment is frequently undertaken by the patient using over-the-counter remedies and without a physician visit or hospital discharge. These difficulties in attaining the ideal set of treatment options for analysis notwithstanding, in most cases a list of hospital treatment options in common use can easily be developed.

Treatment options are expressed as a series of ratios in which the use rate of each treatment is the numerator and the sum of the others is the denominator; this series of computer-generated ratios indicates the relative use by a hospital staff, an HMO, or a clinic practice group of the various treatments available for a disease complex. These are analyzed over the period of a year and in successive years. Such a trend analysis indicates the changing medical response to the same candidate cohort over a period of years. Here is an entity that might be termed "practice style."

Examples. There are about three hundred sets of treatment options (varying from two to fifteen alternative strategies in each set) that govern 75 percent of surgical procedure decision making. A few examples follow.

In *carcinoma of the breast,* the total number of surgical treatment options (total excisional procedures, or TEP) include radical mastectomy (RM), extended radical mastectomy (ERM), modified radical mastectomy (MRM), lumpectomy (LQ), quadrantectomy (QE) with or without lymph node dissection (LNN). Also included are excisional biopsy only (EB) or no excisional procedure (OEP); the latter in turn subsumes a set of radiation/chemotherapy options (R/CT) in most cases. In addition, discharge to another acute-care hospital (out-referral) for special treatment not available locally or discharge for preliminary study, to be followed by later excision as one of the total excisional procedures on a second admission, are programmed. In most hospitals in the United States, the ratio of radical mastectomy to total excisional procedures has undergone a drastic reduction in the last twenty years, and in many community hospitals this change is still going on; it was commenced about 1960 in several teaching centers. For this reason, the total loading factor for the hospital with respect to breast disease is important. This can be given by the ratio of total excisional procedures or total biopsies to total medical/surgical discharges (M/SD). Such vitally important trends are overlooked in the SAV method.

In benign *prostatic obstruction,* the surgical treatment options (including many minor variants) can be grouped together in two aggregates: open prostatectomy (OP) and transurethral prostatectomy (TUR); these can then be expressed as a ratio to other modalities such as antibiotics alone (AA), prolonged catheter drainage (PCD), or discharge without a procedure (DOP). Cystoscopy is a diagnostic procedure whose use in a large candidate cohort is of interest, and it may be used to define a candidate cohort within the group of patients with bladder neck obstruction, as biopsy is used to define a candidate cohort in the universe of patients with breast lumps or abnormalities. The ratio

$$\frac{OP}{(TUR + AA + PCD + DOP)}$$

has been falling in most hospitals over the past two or three decades; it is highest in large referral centers where urologic specialists are referred difficult problem cases either not adapted to transurethral prostatectomy recurring after transurethral prostatectomy. As with any set of treatment option ratios (or corresponding candidate cohort ratios) the ratio of total treatments to total medical/surgical discharges indicates the relative "loading" of that hospital or staff with patients in this category. From such a view of several hospitals, it becomes evident where practice in a specialty is aggregating by referral, usually owing to staffing patterns. This sort of overview of the case-loading and practice patterns in a community is completely missed by the SAV method.

As a third example, consider the treatment options in chronic active *coronary artery disease* (CAD), excluding acute myocardial infarction (AMI). Unlike cystoscopy in bladder neck obstruction, here the diagnostic procedure—coronary catheterization with angiography (CCA)—involves vascular invasion, has its own morbidity and mortality, and should be analyzed as a surgical procedure would be. The professional subgroup doing the procedure (internist, cardiologist, radiologist, surgeon) has no significance in its evaluation or in its categorization (whether or not it is "surgical"). By contrast, its outcome (complications), its frequency in the candidate cohort, and its channel function—bypass is virtually never done without catheterization as a preliminary—make it an extremely important treatment option. In chronic active coronary artery disease, the basic options are cardiac catheter/angiography (CC), bypass (BP), percutaneous angioplasty (APL), out-referral to another acute-care hospital (RAC), or discharge after cardiac catheter/angiography or with none of the above procedures (CCDOT, or DOP). It is of interest that the referral hospitals doing bypass or percutaneous angioplasty handle patients from outside their health services area (HSA) differently than from within their area; the in-referral patients have often been worked up nearer home and therefore have a higher bypass frequency than the local patients, who represent a "natural" mix of CAD patients. Among these treatment options, there are many recent changes; in the past six years the ratio of percutaneous angioplasty to bypass has been rising dramatically and at different rates at different centers, and I am sure there will be other changes as treatments are evolved and perfected in coronary disease. All of these important changes in practice patterns are missed in the SAV method, with its "one shot" look at a single procedure for one year on an uncorrected population base.

Practice Pattern Ratios (TOPPS Ratios)

There are two sets of practice pattern ratios, both of them anticipated in the foregoing analysis and reviewed only briefly here, with ratio examples based on the previous discussion and formulations.

Candidate TOPPS Ratios

Candidate TOPPS ratios are the ratios of the use rate of each treatment option, the sum of all treatment options, or no treatment at all, to the candidate cohort. A set of these ratios for a hospital or clinical practice group indicates the fraction of patients with a set of demand criteria being treated by one of several available treatments. It is analyzed over a period of several years to show annual change. This is the practice pattern (over time) of that hospital, staff, group, HMO, or of an area or population (see below) relating treatment frequency to demand density.

Option Ratios

Option ratios are the ratios of the use of one treatment option to the sum of all other treatment options; these ratios would be identical to the candidate ratios were it not for the fact that in several disease clusters, many patients are sent home without any treatment, studied diagnostically, or referred elsewhere. The option ratios therefore indicate the relative use by a hospital staff of various procedures, the "load factor" for these diseases or their specialists, and the evolution of these use patterns over time. In my experience, option ratios have been strongly influenced by hospital staff, experience, board certification, trustee guidelines, staff customs, and other traditions. There is no reason to expect these ratios to be the same in all areas of a region, a state, or the country as a whole.

Area Complaint Frequencies and Practice Patterns

As mentioned above, complaint frequencies (i.e., symptom density, the size of the candidate cohort) can be related to the population of the area itself, either large or small. The practice pattern ratios can also be aggregated in large or small areas, using zip code aggregates to gain specificity of patient residence regardless of the hospital in which the patient was treated. From such information, one gains an idea not only of the complaint frequency in the area but of the manner in which the medical profession is meeting the demands placed upon it locally. For example, the variability of the complaint frequency of angina pectoris is extremely marked according to affluence, education, and occupation. Such variability is basic to the bypass frequency, is completely overlooked in SAV studies, and cannot be regarded as being due to altered epidemiology of coronary artery disease itself. Complaint frequency is precisely what it is stated to be: the frequency of a certain complaint, the epidemiology of awareness of a symptom that mandates a physician visit (and in our current work, hospitalization). Its density function in turn is a major determinant of the supply of treatment, that is, the treatment frequency.

By analyzing complaint frequencies and practice patterns in all the hospitals treating residents of community XYZ, one gains some insight as to whether the hospitals outside of an area are treating their own local residents differently from those referred in from a greater distance. This is commonplace and should not be overinterpreted or misinterpreted. As already mentioned, a hospital that does coronary bypass and angiography will have a very high procedure rate for referred patients; they have been screened at their local hospitals and sent in specifically for these services. By contrast, local area residents will have a random mix of patients who require less frequent interventional diagnosis or treatment.

Annual Rates and Trend Analysis of TOPPS Ratios

All of the TOPPS ratios (candidate ratios, treatment option ratios, and practice pattern characterizations) must be annualized over time to be understood. The importance of this cannot be overestimated. Remarkable shifts in volume by month or year in small rural hospitals have already been discussed. For example, for the state of Massachusetts as a whole, there were two procedures that underwent a 50 percent change over a two-year period, even in that large area with the same hospitals, the same population, and the same physician mix (19). Were this not to be known, and this type of variability seen between areas, false interpretation might be offered; when such variation is seen to be a function of time, it becomes clear that statistically significant variability in small areas may not be clinically significant. When large annual variability is observed (with the same populations and providers in an area) it is speculation to speak of the small-area variation as due to "practice style."

The Localization of Practice Patterns to Providers

The localization of treatment patterns has been, in my initial experience, entirely to hospitals. Hospital staff homogeneity cannot be assumed, but in the initial development of the TOPPS method and its evaluation, hospitals have been the focus of treatment frequency analysis. The same principles and method can be used for physician groups such as HMOs or private group practice clinics, preferred provider organizations, or individual physicians, with the caveat that for most complex surgical procedures (coronary bypass, hip replacement, extensive cancer surgery, middle ear reconstruction), it is erroneous to localize treatment patterns to a single individual. He (or she) cannot work without the collaboration of a team, often interdisciplinary. It is the team policy that determines the practice pattern ratios. For example, in coronary heart disease this team involves (at the minimum) radiology, medicine (cardiology), anesthesiology, cardiac surgery, and intensive care. Although a single individual may be indentified as the cardiac surgeon, his or her practice pattern is really the net vector of the decision processes of the entire group. When localized to hospitals, aberrancy or regional asymmetries must be reported first to those involved so that analysis, explanation, and in some cases correction, can then be undertaken. To release these data, uncorrected and uninterpretable when expressed as a "small-area variation," only arouses apprehensions and suspicion as to the motives of the research itself.

Small-Area Rates as a Sum of Hospital TOPPS Ratios

The reconstruction of area rates from the summation of individual hospital practices is of interest. Using statewide data bases (such as those now employed at the Massachusetts Health Data Consortium), it is a simple matter to register in the program all patients who live in area XYZ who have had one of a set of treatment options, and to register the regional TOPPS ratios for some specific candidate cohort. This data can then be expressed as an area rate or ratio by simple summation and compared with individual hospital rates, with other comparable areas and other comparable hospitals. In each case, the treatment of "area" residents is included for all hospitals that treat them (inside or outside their own community). When a "small-area rate" is expressed by its hospital makeup, a rational interpretation of regional abnormality can be offered.

TOPPS Ratios: Examples

In the Appendix follow several examples of TOPPS ratios that express treatment frequencies in candidate cohorts (i.e., the demand factor, or patients "at risk" for the procedure) and some examples that express the use of a single treatment option as a function of the relative use of alternative treatments. (These ratios and the terms used in them have been explained in the preceding discussion.) All of these ratios and expressions are designed for use in a large or statewide data base, employing the ICDA-9 code, and in some cases, using DRG and MCD categories for aggregation or clarification. Terms are redefined only when the foregoing paragraphs did not cover them adequately. Except where indicated otherwise (e.g., populations), the units both in the numerator and denominator are numbers of hospital discharges of that class or set in a given year. In all cases, the same ratios are to be calculated for successive years. The ratios can apply to specific hospitals, or to areas (i.e., geographically defined population groups). The area rates can be calculated directly from patient residence or by aggregating the hospitals treating patients from that area. Several of these ratios can be plotted against cost, outcome, length of stay, and other indices, so as to compare the work of various hospitals or the services given in various areas.

OTHER INDICES OF ACCESS AND OF PUBLIC SERVICE

Access versus Excess, "Available" versus "Enough"

One of the enigmas of surgical care in this country and of the triage of surgical patients has to do with the widespread availability of certain surgical, complex, or invasive medical technologies. In many instances, local communities are anxious to have this capability locally available (e.g., cardiac surgery, ultrasonography, NMR, total hip replacement). It is an ethnocentric source of pride for their community if their "own hospital" can provide these services. On the other hand, when these services are made available to small communities or in outlying areas, or in small hospitals in close juxtaposition to established centers, they may be done by physicians who are not fully trained, who are not supported by an adequate interdisciplinary team, and who do not have a "critical mass" of candidates to deal with these patients in an ideal way.

Using the TOPPS method of analyzing treatment options and practice profiles, it is possible to look at total volume in relation to outcome not only of procedures, but also for candidate cohorts after distribution to specific hospitals and areas. In-transfer and out-transfer become very important and are readily handled if the data set has been properly designed and programmed. For example, in the treatment of acute myocardial infarction, transfer to a major center within forty-eight hours is often a sign of excellent care and of the triage selection of very sick patients for transfer to a center where angiography, bypass, and angioplasty are available. On superficial judgment, and without a regional set of TOPPS ratios, such a hospital might be considered as accepting only mild AMI cases for treatment and sending them home prematurely. In point of fact, they are demonstrating a triage and referral model of practice that should ideally characterize all community hospitals. Judgments of this type can be offered only if treatment pattern ratios are completed for a disease complex for a large area and its constituent smaller areas, including the work of all hospitals caring for residents of that area as well as nearby out-of-state hospitals.

Are Difficult Cases Avoided?
Why Do Experts Sometimes Show a High Mortality?

It is a familiar phenomenon in American medicine that many hospitals do not wish to take care of patients with severe cerebrovascular injuries, patients with certain types of crippling due to congenital disease, and patients with certain types of chronic brain disease and trauma. These patients are often "dumped" on some center, frequently a tax-supported hospital that may be remote from their residence.

Analogous problems exist in surgery with particular reference to burns, complex late vascular reconstruction for distal gangrene (particularly in diabetes), multiple severe fractures in very elderly people, and inoperable or dimly operable congenital anomalies in the newborn (such as spina bifida). In evaluating the surgical services available to an area, it is therefore important to inquire as to what disposition is being made for cases such as these. Is there a local facility, sometimes a veterans' hospital, that can deal with them at an acceptable standard of specialist care? Are they being dumped as "welfare cases" in some tax-supported hospital? Are they being kept in a local hospital until their insurance runs out and then dumped elsewhere? These and other difficult questions of surgical care availability in areas can be evaluated using the TOPPS method, applying it without bias to all the hospitals in a region or area.

With accumulation of difficult cases as a referral function, the center with the greatest expertise may exhibit a high mortality or morbidity, the specialist there being willing to take on difficult cases not accepted for treatment elsewhere.

OUTCOMES AND COST

Using TOPPS ratios either for candidate cohorts or treatment options, a comparative study can be made of outcomes. Such a study relates these outcomes to the use of specific procedures for a specific set of candidates, and to a comparison among alternative procedures either within a hospital or among several hospitals. My experience in arranging such outcome programs is confined to in-hospital data and does not include later judgments as to clinical effectiveness. With this limitation, outcome can be based on length of stay, complications, secondary corrective procedures, and mortality.

Similarly, in the case of costs (charges) to the payer, data can be aggregated as a function either of candidate or of option ratios. In our data base, these data on costs and charges are available since 1983. Without localization to hospitals, such data would be neither collectible or interpretable. Once aggregated, however, regional, statewide, or community expenditures for the use of several alternative procedures in a specific candidate cohort can be calculated and meaningful comparisons made.

Although some sort of cost-benefit analysis might be done on comparative complication rates or mortalities expressed on a cost basis for several alternative treatments, it is unwise to estimate cost-benefit ratios in the absence of late follow-up, cure rates, or rehabilitation scores.

For the interpretation of costs and case-loading, some sort of severity index would be invaluable to distinguish the more expensive high-risk complex clinical challenges ("high-cost users") from the simpler cases (23). A day-rating scale has been suggested (23), a complex grid of comorbidities has been advanced (24), and the use of simple identifiers such as emergency admission or the necessity of blood transfusion has been suggested (25). All three of these methods show promise and can be used with the TOPPS method to segregate treatment candidates according to severity. This makes possible the interpretation of costs and outcomes on a realistic basis.

APPENDIX

Derivation of a few TOPPS ratios for several disease entities are shown here as examples. The reader is referred to the text for the key to the abbreviations used.

A. Carcinoma of the Breast

1. Frequency of operation in relation to total biopsy
   $$\frac{TEP}{TBx}$$
2. Frequency of modified radical mastectomy among positive biopsies
   $$\frac{MRM}{CaBx}$$
3. Frequency of radical mastectomy among all operative procedures
   $$\frac{RM}{TEP}$$
4. Positivity fraction of biopsies
   $$\frac{CaBx}{TBx}$$
5. Surgical treatment as a fraction of all other treatments
   $$\frac{TEP}{(EB + OEP + R/CT)}$$
6. Loading factor for breast disease in the hospital (M/SD = Total Medical and Surgical Discharges)
   $$\frac{BBx}{M/SD}$$
7. Population complaint frequency for region or area XYZ
   $$\frac{BBx}{Pop\ XYZ}$$
8. Radical mastectomy for a region by (n) hospitals (for residents of area XYZ)
   $$RM_{XYZ} = (RM)\ Hosp\ A + (RM)\ Hosp\ B + \ldots (RM)\ Hosp\ n$$

All the above ratios may be stratified by age, prior cancer (e.g., other breast), subsequent radiotherapy or chemotherapy, and plotted for covariance analysis against outcomes.

B. Hysterectomy
1. Frequency of operation in a candidate cohort (all ratios may be expressed for a hospital or community)

$$\frac{\text{HYST}}{\text{TGD}}$$

2. In a refined candidate cohort

$$\frac{\text{HYST}}{[\text{TGD} - (\text{DCA} + \text{MING})]}$$

3. Frequency of hysterectomy versus certain other alternatives

$$\frac{\text{HYST}}{(\text{D\&C}_A + \text{TGD}_{DOT})}$$

C. Cesarean Section
1. Frequency of cesarean section (in third trimester pregnancy)

$$\frac{\text{CS}}{\text{TLB}}$$

or

$$\frac{\text{CS}}{\text{TLB} - \text{CS}} = \frac{\text{CS}}{\text{TPD}}$$

As in other ratios, these can be stratified for age and clinical factors (primiparity, prior cesarean); and ratios of all the hospitals can be plotted as covariance functions for cost, professional fees, maternal morbidity (LOS, complications), and fetal outcome (mortality, LOS, neonatal ICU).

D. Prostatectomy
1. Frequency of prostatectomy in a candidate cohort

$$\frac{\text{OP} + \text{TUR}}{(\text{PH} + \text{BNO} + \text{OU})}$$

2. Relative frequency of the use of transurethral prostatectomy compared with other alternatives

$$\frac{\text{TUR}}{(\text{OP} + \text{AA} + \text{PCD} + \text{DOP})}$$

E. Coronary Heart Disease
   1. Candidate cohort for chronic artery disease (CAD), excluding AMI, consists of the six primary (CHD_6) codes plus the five secondary (SEC_5) subsets that require "marker" identification
   $$CAD = (CHD_6 + SEC_5)$$
   2. Frequency of cardiac catheterization in candidate cohort
   $$\frac{CC}{(CHD_6 + SEC_5)}$$

The above ratios can be expressed for each hospital, summed for hospitals, or programmed to give the rate for any area, either directly from patients' residence, or as an aggregate of all hospitals treating patients from that area; the same is true of the following ratios.

   3. Frequency of bypass in candidate cohort
   $$\frac{BP}{(CHD_6 + SEC_5)}$$
   of angioplasty
   $$\frac{APL}{(CHD_6 - SEC_5)}$$
   4. Relative use of angioplasty
   $$\frac{APL}{BP}$$
   5. Frequency of total coronary intervention (can be calculated for CAD or AMI)
   $$\frac{(APL + BP)}{CHD_6 + SEC_5}$$
   or
   $$\frac{APL + BP}{AMI}$$

F. Expressions for Hospitals and Areas (General Terms)

When programming for residents of area XYZ in whatever hospital they are treated, then the following ratios can be used:

1. Treatment frequency for a hospital

$$\frac{\text{Procedure}}{\text{Candidate Cohort}}$$

2. The area complaint frequency or symptom density (i.e., frequency of hospitalization for that system or disease complex)

$$\frac{\Sigma \text{ (Candidate Cohorts)} \begin{matrix}\text{Hosp A} \\ \text{Hosp } n\end{matrix}}{\text{Pop XYZ}}$$

3. Area treatment frequency

$$\frac{\Sigma \text{ (Procedures)} \begin{matrix}\text{Hosp A} \\ \text{Hosp } n\end{matrix}}{\text{Pop XYZ}}$$

The above ratios provide the "small-area rate" parsed according to the work of each hospital.

4. Area ratio of treatment frequency to candidate cohort

$$\frac{\Sigma \text{ (Procedure)} \begin{matrix}\text{Hosp A} \\ \text{Hosp } n\end{matrix}}{\Sigma \text{ (Candidate Cohort)} \begin{matrix}\text{Hosp A} \\ \text{Hosp } n\end{matrix}}$$

The above numerator and denominator subsets include all residents of area XYZ wherever they are treated.

REFERENCES

1. Wennberg, J.E., and Gittelsohn, A.M. Small-area variations in health care delivery. *Science* 182:1102–8 (1973).
2. Lewis, C.L. Variations in the incidence of surgery. *N Eng J Med* 281:880–83 (1969).
3. Moore, E.D. Small-area variations studies: Illuminating or misleading? *Health Affairs* 4:96–101 (1985).
4. McPherson, K. Regional variations in health care: Small-area variation studies and longitudinal outcome studies. *International Newsletter on Regional Variations in Health Care* 1:2 (1986).
5. See the series of articles in *Health Affairs* 3,2 (1984).
6. Lewis, C.E. Variations in the incidence of surgery. *N Eng J Med* 281:880–83 (1969).
7. Rothberg, D.L. *Regional Variations in Hospital Use: Geographic and Temporal Patterns of Care in the United States.* Lexington and Toronto: Lexington Books (1982).
8. Wennberg, J.E., and Gittelsohn, A.M. Health care delivery in Maine: 1: Patterns of use of common surgical procedures. *J Maine Med Assoc* 66:123 (1975).
9. Wennberg, J.E. Gittelsohn, A.M., and Shapiro, N. Health care delivery in Maine. 3: Evaluating the level of hospital performance. *J Maine Med Assoc* 66:11 (1975).
10. Brook, R.H., Lohr, K., Chassin, M., et al. Geographic variations in the use of services: Do they have any clinical significance? *Health Affairs* 3:63–73 (1984).
11. Moore, F.D. Small-area variations in health care delivery: A critique. *J Maine Med Assoc* 68:49–52 (1977).
12. Moore, F.D. Variations in the use of medical and surgical services. *N Eng J Med* 315:649–50 (1986).
13. Gittelsohn, A.M., and Wennberg, J.E. The authors respond. *J Maine Med Assoc* 68:53–57 (1977).
14. Caper, P., and Spitzer, M. In defense of small-area analysis. *Health Affairs* 4:115–19 (1985).
15. Wennberg, J.E. To the editor. *N Eng J Med* 315:650 (1986).
16. Hinkle, L.E. Occupation, education, and coronary heart disease. *Science* 161:238–46 (1968).
17. Wennberg, J.E., McPherson, K., and Caper, P. Will payment based on diagnosis-related groups control hospital costs? *N Eng J Med* 311:295–300 (1984).
18. Wennberg, J.E. Dealing with medical practice variations: A proposal for action. *Health Affairs* 3:6–32 (1984).
19. Donahue, C.L., Barnes, B.A., and O'Brien, E. *Variations in Surgical Utilization in Massachusetts.* Boston: Health Planning Council of Greater Boston (1984).
20. Wennberg, J.E., and Gittelsohn, A.M. Variations in medical care among small areas. *Scientific American,* 246:120–33 (1982).

21. Wennberg, J.E. Which rate is right? *N Eng J Med* 314:310–11 (1986).
22. Moore, F.D., and Pratt, L.W. Tonsillectomy in Maine: Regulation versus education as modulators of medical care. *Ann Surg* 194:232–41 (1981).
23. Zook, C.J., and Moore, F.D. High-cost users of medical care. *N Eng J Med* 302.996–1002 (1980).
24. Horn, S.D., and Horn, R.A. Reliability and validity of the severity of illness index. *Med Care* 24:159–78 (1986).
25. Munoz, E., Regan, D.M., Margolis, I.B., and Wise, L. Surgonomics: The identifier concept. *Ann Surg* 202:119–25 (1985).

6 Managing Surgical Admissions

Leslie L. Roos, Ph.D., and Noralou P. Roos, Ph.D.

It is generally acknowledged that the hospital sector absorbs the largest proportion of expenditures on health care. Because an individual's health status has been shown repeatedly to be the best predictor of hospitalization (1), pressures for expansion of this sector are expected to increase dramatically over the next several decades with the growth in the numbers of elderly—the frailest, most needy group in the population (2).

Predictions of an increasing burden on hospitals have generally ignored an important determinant of utilization—the hospitalization practices of the individual physician. Most studies have investigated determinants of utilization without regard to the context (both the availability of hospital beds and physician discretion) in which services are received (3). However, small-area variations in surgical and hospitalization rates have been found to be relatively unrelated to variations in the health status of area residents (4–5). These studies take border-crossing into account and have found these variations in utilization across many medical and surgical conditions (6–9).

Some small-area rates of hospitalization for certain medical and surgical conditions have been shown to vary much more than others. Typical of high-variation conditions are atherosclerosis, disorders of the biliary tract, peptic ulcer, and tonsillectomy. Similar variations have been found for many conditions between countries with very different ways of organizing their health care systems. Hence the generalization that "only a small proportion of hospitalizations fit a model based on medical need" (3).

We gratefully acknowledge the help of the Manitoba Health Services Commission. The initial draft of this chapter was supported by the Review of Demography and Its Implications for Economic and Social Policy, Health and Welfare, Canada. This research was supported by National Health Research and Development Project No. 6607-1187-44 and by Career Scientist Award No. 6607-1314-48. Interpretations and viewpoints contained in this chapter are our own and do not necessarily represent the opinion of either the Manitoba Health Services Commission or Health and Welfare Canada.

Managing the discretionary component in hospital admissions is both very difficult and of central importance for cost savings (10–11). Physicians are responsible for decisions that govern how a large proportion of each health care dollar is spent (12). Although hospital costs have been rising more rapidly than the overall rate of inflation (13), little attention has been paid to the gatekeeper role of physicians. To date, most attention has focused either on the implications of high technology for costs or on elderly individuals' use of care resources and the projected expansion of the numbers of the very old over the next several decades.

While the elderly, particularly the very elderly (those eighty-five years and older), do use many more hospital days than others, there are comparatively few of them, so their total impact on the health care system seems much less than the impact of the practices of certain physicians. Thus, a projected 10 percent increase in the numbers of very elderly in Manitoba, for example, might lead to increased consumption of approximately 16,000 hospital days; a 10 percent increase in physicians who are prone to hospitalize their patients would result in 45,000 additional hospital days (14).

If variations in physicians' hospitalization styles are both as large as suggested and substantially independent of patient need, these findings would have important implications for health planners. Physicians' practice styles (particularly when they reflect professional uncertainty) can be changed (15); patient "need" is much less susceptible to change. If utilization is based on need, then restrictions on health care spending imply rationing. If need can be met with more cost-effective medicine, then rationing does not become an issue (3).

The Rand Health Insurance Experiment has demonstrated that programs to reduce unnecessary use of health care that target the consumer-patient (e.g., copayment schemes) work in pernicious ways. Copayment markedly reduced utilization of health care services by the poor and also reduced the use of all kinds of medical care, not just that considered unnecessary or inappropriate (16). Clearly, efforts to ensure that medical care is delivered in the most cost-effective way must look at the medical profession. The identification of causes of hospital admission that are highly discretionary across widely divergent geographic areas emphasizes the need to focus on such data.

PHYSICIANS' PRACTICE STYLES

Few direct studies of the influence of physicians' practices on hospitalization patterns exist. Interviews with physicians and case studies provide anecdotal examples of the influence of physicians' varied styles on hospital utilization patterns (17–18). Rosenblatt and Moscovice attempted to identify directly the nonmedical factors affecting the rate at which physicians hospitalize ambulatory patients (19). But this study and others reviewed by Eisenberg did not control directly for disease severity or patient case mix (20).

Connell, Blide, and Hanken reported that physicians practicing in areas with high hospitalization rates for diabetes were more likely to admit patients who were mildly ill than were their counterparts practicing in low-rate areas (21). However, earlier Manitoba research found no such relationship between physicians standards of selecting cases for tonsillectomy and small-area rates of surgery (22). Although many researchers assume that significant differences in physicians' practice patterns are the primary reason for small-area variations in hospitalization rates (23), critics argue that the importance of practice styles in determining these variations must be studied directly (24–26).

Evidence of marked differences in physicians' practice styles comes from several sources. The influence of physicians' styles on lengths of stay has recently been compared with that of severity of illness within the diagnosis-related groups (DRGs) used for American Medicare payments. Practice variation accounted for more of the variance in lengths of stay than did severity of illness (27).

Physicians in prepaid groups (health maintenance organizations) have long been thought to have a less hospital-intensive style than that of the average physician. Although skeptics have criticized the atypical enrollment pattern of these groups and the failure to describe out-of-plan usage adequately, the data are intriguing (28). Roch, Evans, and Pascoe noted that Manitobans are hospitalized at a rate in excess of twice that to be expected if they were members of a health maintenance organization such as the Kaiser-Permanente medical plan.

Physician opinions about the need for surgery have been found to differ in several types of studies. About 25 percent of the patients for whom surgery is recommended have that opinion reversed if a second surgeon is consulted (30). Doctors asked to rate the appropriateness of a large number of indicators for performing six common procedures disagreed markedly (31). Physicians evaluating hypothetical cases on a patient's need for hospitalization or surgery also demonstrated divergence of opinion (32–35). However, responses to hypothetical cases may not reflect actual practices. Ontario surgeons in counties with high rates for particular procedures were not more likely to opt for surgical treatment in a hypothetical case than surgeons in counties with low rates; disagreements occurred in all counties regardless of their rates (36).

A Manitoba study of changes in surgical workload and patient utilization provides direct evidence on the impact of physician discretion (8). Individual physician workloads remained fairly stable over time when a new surgically active physician moved into an area, while population utilization increased markedly. When such physicians left an area, the surgical workloads of the remaining physicians increased significantly while population utilization stayed essentially the same. Both physician workload and surgical utilization in control areas increased gradually over the period studied. Data on individual procedures, as well as overall figures, emphasized the importance of physician discretion.

In the absence of uniform policy across hospitals, considerable discretion also exists with regard to ambulatory surgery. Between 1974 and 1983, the number of procedures performed as same-day surgery in Canada increased from 55,340 to 122,244, an increase of 121 percent. Approximately 80 percent of the American public prefers ambulatory surgery to inpatient care for minor procedures (37). When feasible, outpatient surgery may be the site of choice for elderly patients, given the adverse affects of enforced bed rest and change from a customary environment (38).

Syracuse, New York, a metropolitan area with relatively few acute-care beds (3.0 per 1,000 people), performed 37 percent of all hospital-based surgery on an ambulatory basis in 1983. This rate is considerably higher than that recorded elsewhere (39). In the past, many surgeons were unwilling to change practice patterns, preferring to admit patients to a hospital for three days than to use an ambulatory surgery approach (40). However, preadmission review in the United States has put considerable pressure upon physicians to perform same-day surgery.

UNCERTAINTY AND DISCRETION

Several sources of professional uncertainty in diagnosing illness and prescribing treatment have been identified. (1) There are often difficulties in classifying a patient so that the probabilities of existence of disease, prognosis, and treatment outcomes can be reasonably ascertained. (2) Information on the probabilities of treatment outcome under controlled circumstances may not exist. (3) Even when patients are appropriately classified and outcome probabilities are known, the utilities that patients attach to different outcomes may be unknown by the physician (3, 41–42).

Variation in rates of admission may be affected both by professional uncertainty about the efficacy of a procedure and by discretion as to whether a relatively minor procedure is done on an outpatient basis.

Considerable disagreement exists over the effectiveness of various treatments such as tonsillectomy, knee operations, and back and neck surgery. As discussed below, some surgical procedures with the highest variation (tubal interruptions, dental extractions, etc.) are routinely performed by many (but not all) hospitals on an outpatient basis. Physician discretion also determines whether patients with specific conditions require admission to hospital or can be handled on a "watch-and-wait-and-report-new-developments-to-the-physician" basis. In similar fashion, differing physician practice patterns likely account for the high variation in admission rates for such medical conditions as pediatric pneumonia, pediatric bronchitis and asthma, chest pain, and peptic ulcer.

RESEARCH NEEDS

This chapter suggests several ways to categorize hospitals and physicians according to the extent that patients are hospitalized in situations where other institutions and providers might not do so. Extensive effort is needed to develop these indices further, to test their validity and generalizability, and to determine their usefulness to those managing the health care sector. Each index takes the statistically accepted approach of generating counts of individuals hospitalized (the *observed* figure) and comparing these counts with the figure that would be expected for the institution or provider being considered (the *expected* figure).

The data bases cited here have been developed from claims filed routinely by hospitals and physicians with the government agency responsible for administering the insured medical and hospital services in Manitoba. When used appropriately, the data can provide an accurate and reliable representation of health care utilization (43–44). For the most part, the measures described in this chapter use hospital information on procedures; coding for procedures is generally more reliable than that for diagnostic information (45–46). The diagnostic coding we used followed the DRG framework (47), but was more conservative, combining categories when the number of cases was small.

The Measurement of Discretion in Hospital Admissions

The discretion in hospital admissions (DHA) measure has been developed from American data on variation in medical and surgical causes of hospital admission. This index builds on the diagnosis-related group (DRG) method of classifying patients into groups characterized by resource consumption once admitted to hospital (47–48).

The consistency in variation in admission rates of similar patients across areas has been used to develop an index reflecting the profession's discretion/uncertainty as to whether a patient "needs" to be hospitalized (49). Development of the DHA measure starts with the proportion of a hospital's patients whose DRGs place them in the discretionary (high-variation) admission category. Adjusting for age and sex, this observed figure can be compared with the proportion expected for this hospital (on the basis of provincial norms). Since the observed/expected ratio will be 1.0 for the geographic unit as a whole, ratios greater than 1.0 indicate more discretionary admissions than expected.

The basic logic of this measure can be applied to either hospital or physician data. DHAs for separate services (surgical and medical) could be easily developed. The measure seems more suited for work with hospitals than with physicians; individual physicians might hospitalize very few patients, but if their hospitalizations involved DRGs in the high-variation categories, they would have high scores on this measure. This DHA index should allow peer-review bodies, hospital administrators, and reimbursement agencies to determine which hospitals (and physicians) admit disproportionate numbers of patients with conditions for which widespread disagreement exists about the necessity for acute hospital care.

The Measurement of Ambulatory Surgery Utilization

To date, measures describing the amount of variation in the use of outpatient surgery across hospitals and across physicians within hospitals have been lacking. Such data can help develop firm estimates of the potential for increased outpatient usage as well as the appropriate target for efforts to change utilization patterns. Such attention to outpatient surgery is highlighted by an examination of surgical admissions having the highest variation. Counting only inpatient admissions in the data base, the thirteen categories of surgical admissions producing very high variation scores are procedures routinely performed by many hospitals on an outpatient basis (50).

An index of ambulatory surgery utilization (the ASU measure) has been developed, identifying those procedures most commonly done on an ambulatory basis (39). Procedures were included when performed in both inpatient and outpatient settings in Manitoba. To be considered, these procedures could not be performed more than 85 percent of the time in one setting; to emphasize the potential for substitution, only inpatient cases discharged within three days of admission were compared with the outpatient surgery cases.

The ASU measure has been produced in a way similar to that described above for the DHA measure. An age- and sex-adjusted expected number of outpatient surgeries based on provincial norms and each hospital's (or physician's) current surgical case mix was generated. The hospital's (or physician's) observed number was divided by this expected number to give an observed/expected ratio. With 1.0 being the provincial average, comparisons among institutions and providers were easily made.

The Measurement of Physician Hospitalization Style

The physician hospitalization style (PHS) measure used Manitoba claims data to describe physicians' hospitalization styles after adjusting for case-mix characteristics of their primary patients (51). To describe the PHS index in more depth, patients were uniquely assigned to that physician (general or family practitioner, internist, general surgeon, or obstetrician/gynecologist) seen most frequently over each of two two-year periods (1972–74 and 1974–76). Four indices were developed including (1) percentage of primary patients hospitalized; (2) mean number of readmissions for such patients; (3) mean length of stay; and (4) total days of hospitalization per primary care patient (a summary measure combining the first three). Rates of admission, not length of stay, were shown to be strongly related to this summary measure. Marked variations in the hospitalization indices were observed across physicians; these variations could not be explained by the health or sociodemographic characteristics of a physician's patients.

Generalizability and Stability

Information on hospital and physician practice seems likely to be applicable across adult age groups. Other research on physician and hospital determinants of complications following surgery has found similar variables relevant to understanding utilization of younger and older adult patients (52–53). To assure generalizability of the work, ongoing Manitoba analyses will use both all adults and just those sixty-five years of age and over. However, there is a special need to study physicians' practice styles among one group of elderly—those who receive care immediately preceding death. Much of the health care utilization of the very old appears to be associated with dying rather than with aging per se, with a large portion of expenditures occurring in the last few months prior to death (54–56). Given the magnitude of these expenditures, a special focus on practice style and this group is warranted.

None of the indices suggested has been studied over a considerable period of time. The PHS (physician hospitalization style) measure is reasonably stable over the short term (for a pair of adjacent two-year periods, the Pearson's r ranged from .59 to .70). Certain aspects of a physician's practice—such as the volume and type of surgical procedures performed—have been shown to be quite consistent over time (53). Without new technologies or special interventions, such practice characteristics normally change slowly in response to professional opinion, personal interests, and so forth.

Surgical causes of hospital admission tend to be reasonably stable in each medical market area; for example, areas with high population-based rates of prostatectomy one year would tend to have similar rates the next year (3). Since the DHA measure has been derived from aggregating such differing causes of admission from four different states, considerable stability over time would be expected.

Further development needs to consider both the measures' short-term stability (reliability) and their longer-term consistency. After confidence in the measures has been established, demonstration projects and other interventions can try to alter the care being given in cost-effective ways. Successful interventions would presumably lead to changes measurable by these indices.

Practice Style, Quality of Care, and Patient Outcomes

Discretionary hospital admissions also have implications for quality of care. Hospitalizations are not always in the patients' best interest; the high risk of hospital-acquired infections and falls in the elderly patient suggests that quite the opposite may be true (57). Furthermore, physicians practicing in areas with high admission rates for diabetes mellitus (a very high-variation cause of admission) were found to provide lower quality of care for this condition (patients underwent less thorough testing) than did physicians working in areas with low hospital admission rates (21). Similarly, research on hysterectomy rates in Saskatchewan found that a reduction in admissions for hysterectomy (a high-variation procedure) was associated with a drop in the proportion of cases judged "unjustified" by a professional committee set up to study this procedure (58).

As noted above, analyses of health status have shown no significant differences between high- and low-utilization areas. Doing such studies for areas whose residents tend to be hospitalized more or less frequently for discretionary reasons, or for areas whose residents disproportionately receive inpatient or outpatient surgery, would be relatively easy. The availability of Manitoba Health Services Commission data in conjunction with extensive health status data from interviews of elderly Manitobans conducted in 1971, 1976, and 1983 would permit such research (59–60).

Convincing hospitals and physicians that changes in practice style need not affect quality of care probably depends upon more direct evidence. Individual patients must be able to be assigned to physicians (and hospitals) initially, and then followed over a period of time. To keep the logic of the argument, individual patients must stay with the same physician (or hospital) throughout the time in which they are followed. The length of follow-up should be at least ten years to give any differences in the quality of care time to develop.

Research on the PHS measure counted visits during a two-year period for patient assignment to particular physicians (51). Using such successive two-year blocks over a ten-year period would measure how many individuals consistently visit the same physician. Given the many patients who visit a physician infrequently, five-year periods might be preferred. A patient having the same doctor as his primary physician during the two adjacent five-year periods (assuming a ten-year study) would enter into the study.

Undertaking such analyses with a large enough sample would permit the investigation of specific medical conditions (angina, hypertension, diabetes, etc.) where outcomes might differ after treatment by physicians whose practice styles were high and low on this "hospitalization-prone" dimension. Depending on the medical condition and on the particular information in the data base, certain characteristics of the care can be specified (surgery, ambulatory visits, diagnostic tests).

Large claims data bases are good at identifying such outcomes as

—mortality
—readmissions to the same or a different hospital
—admissions to nursing homes
—patients needing home care services
—patients diagnosed with particular other conditions.

A literature is developing as to how to do such outcome research with minimal biases (53, 61, 62). Thus direct comparisons of long-term outcomes of patients of physicians with different hospitalization styles could be made, controlling for such variables as physician specialty. As noted, survey-based measures of health status can be linked with the claims data; 1983 health-status measures can be compared for individuals having physicians with differing degrees of "hospital proneness."

DISCUSSION

Existing health care systems may well be able to adapt to increased numbers of elderly without expanding acute-care beds. In Manitoba, despite an increase in the numbers of elderly in the 1970s (age- and sex-specific projections predicted an 8.3 percent increase in utilization between 1970 and 1981), the number of hospital days used by the Manitoba population actually decreased 6.3 percent per 1,000 people (29). This decrease reflected an administrative decision to reduce the numbers of hospital beds in certain areas. A similar pattern was found in British Columbia, where acute hospital usage fell markedly in the 1970s despite a rapidly aging population (63). Thus the health care system is potentially malleable. Manitoba built nursing home beds in the 1970s and currently plans to increase capacity for "not-for-admission surgery" and home care as alternatives to expanding the acute-care sector.

The relationships among measures can give an idea of the ease with which change can be brought about. Do "hospitalization-prone" physicians (high on the PHS measure) disproportionately admit patients having the high-variation diagnoses? What is the diagnostic mix of patients admitted by "nonhospitalization-prone" physicians? Do "hospitalization-prone" physicians tend to practice in hospitals high on the DHA measure? If patients admitted to hospital by "hospitalization-prone" physicians are those with diagnoses for which little professional consensus on the need for hospitalization exists, modifying physician behavior through feedback may be quite possible (6, 25).

The indices presented here have considerable potential in facilitating cost control without negatively affecting the quality of care. For example, the DHA measure could be used in several ways; hospitals facing bed shortages could undertake a review of admissions over the past three months. What number of bed days were used by patients admitted with high-variation diagnoses? Hospital utilization committees could pull a random sample of charts and assess the degree to which these admissions were necessary. What procedures could have been performed on an outpatient basis? Meetings with medical staff might focus on the general problem of bed shortages and develop specific guidelines for admission for high-variation categories. Individual physicians who generally admit patients in high-variation DRGs or who score high on the ASU measure could be identified; their practice styles could subsequently be monitored. When such guidelines were developed for the high-variation procedure tonsillectomy in Vermont and Pittsburgh, tonsillectomy at the two demonstration hospitals fell markedly (64–65).

Insurers might also want to know which hospitals have higher than expected admission rates for high-variation procedures. Analysis might focus either on very high and high causes of admissions overall or on specific causes of admission. Roos, Wennberg, and McPherson identified several medical causes of admission that are both highly variable and have high resource requirements (49). In particular, hospital admissions for chronic obstructive lung disease and for pediatric pneumonia are heavily reimbursed under the U.S. prospective payment system. Table 6.1 summarizes data on consistency and variation in hospitalization rates (49).

Having several measures is important because of the number of ways in which health care resources can be spent. As Wennberg, McPherson, and Caper stressed, a hospital serving a given area may have a short length of stay for patients in a given DRG but a large number of patients hospitalized for this DRG (11). Another hospital may tend to admit patients who are being treated on an outpatient or ambulatory basis elsewhere. Such multiple measures are particularly important for urban teaching hospitals where constructing small market areas is difficult because of border-crossing within metropolitan areas and referrals from other regions.

These measures are relevant for efforts at cost control across different political systems. Insurers, both in the United States and elsewhere, are increasingly interested in the provision of services without hospitalization. In a political system using "global" budgets to control hospital costs (such as Canada and many European countries), hospitals may have great difficulties staying within their budgets. Funding agencies are likely to wish to monitor hospital performance and feedback information on how a given hospital might reduce its expenditures.

CONCLUSION

Although this chapter has concentrated on discretionary hospitalization, other measures of physician and hospital behavior are either in use or under development. Analysis of diagnosis-related groups is well established as part of the American Medicare system (47–48). As noted above, small-area analyses are being carried out by researchers and policy analysts in a number of countries. Ongoing work suggests the possibilities of incorporating analyses of hospital readmissions into quality control and cost-of-care studies (52, 66). Thus a diversity of approaches are available for the health care analyst.

All the methods suggested to reduce admissions of patients in high-variation categories have focused on the medical profession and its

TABLE 6.1. Classification of Modified DRG Categories by Degree of Variation in Hospitalization Rate

Medical Causes of Admission	Surgical Causes of Admission
Low Variation	*Low Variation*
*Acute myocardial infarction	*Inguinal and femoral hernia operation
*Specific cerebrovascular disorder	*Major small and large bowel operation
	Gallbladder disorders with cholecystectomy
	*Hip repair except joint replacement
Moderate Variation	*Moderate Variation*
*Gastrointestinal hemorrhage	Appendicitis with appendectomy
High Variation	*High Variation*
*Urinary tract stones	Hysterectomy
Digestive malignancy	Major joint operations
*Syncope and collapse	Major cardiovascular operations
Heart failure and shock	Other adult hernia operations
*Respiratory neoplasms	Anal operations
Seizures and headaches	Soft tissue operations
Angina pectoris	*Lens operations
Toxic effects of drugs	Foot operations
*Cardiac arrhythmias	Transurethral operations
G.I. obstruction	
*Adult simple pneumonias	
Miscellaneous injuries to extremities	
Very High 1	*Very High 1*
Kidney and urinary tract infections	Back and neck operations
Adult gastroenteritis	Hand operations except ganglion
*Medical back problems	Knee operations
Circulatory disorders excluding AMI, with cardiac catheterization	
Red blood cell disorders	
Cellulitis	
Adult diabetes	
Very High 2	*Very High 2*
*Chest pain	Tonsillectomy
Deep vein thrombophlebitis	Extraocular operations
*Acute adjustment reaction	Miscellaneous ear, nose, and throat operations
*Adult otitis media and URI	*Other T & A operations
Respiratory signs and symptoms	D & C, conization except for malignancy
Chronic obstructive lung disease	
Trauma to skin, subcutaneous tissue, and breast	Breast biopsy and local excision for nonmalignancy
Adult bronchitis and asthma	
*Hypertension	*Other female laparoscopic operations
*Pediatric gastro-enteritis	*Tubal interruptions for nonmalignancy
*Peptic ulcer	
*Pediatric bronchitis and pneumonia	*Dental extractions and restorations
*Organic mental syndromes	*Laparoscopic tubal interruption
*Atherosclerosis	
*Pediatric otitis media and URI	
*Pediatric pneumonia	
*Chemotherapy	

* These DRG groups have variation scores within two decile ranks across four states. All categories above show consistency in variation scores across at least three states.

regulators, rather than on the patient. Some physicians clearly believe strongly in the effectiveness of hospital treatment for a given condition, while others, no doubt equally strongly, believe it inappropriate or unnecessary to hospitalize patients with this condition. Who is right needs to be addressed both by the physician community and by policymakers. Where the data do not permit resolution, the profession needs to collaborate in research to resolve these critical questions. At the same time, given the pressures for cost control, insurers and policy-making bodies need to push actively for programs moving certain services out of the hospital.

From a broader perspective, what are the alternatives to the status quo projected into the future? Physicians have a great deal of discretion in influencing

—the number and type of services to be provided by the physician himself
—the number and type of services to be provided to the patient by the rest of the health care system

This overview has addressed only costs placed upon the hospital system as a result of physician discretion. As Lomas, Stoddart, and Barer stressed, explicit consideration must be given "to alternative ways of structuring the inputs of the health care production process" (67). Increased efficiency becomes a necessity. The various possibilities include

—moving some categories of medical and surgical treatment to an outpatient or ambulatory setting
—reducing rates of particular therapies (such as some common surgical procedures)
—reducing length of stay for some DRGs
—developing and implementing cost-containment measures for ambulatory care

The measures discussed in this chapter can be used to help address increased use of outpatient and ambulatory treatments. Considerable activity currently focuses on small-area variation and length-of-stay issues; ambulatory care needs more research attention. As noted in chapter 2 above, efforts also need to be directed toward such longer-term issues as the physician surplus and its implications for cost containment.

APPENDIX

The indices measuring hospital admissions (DHA and ASU) have been designed to permit adjustment for possible age and sex differences among hospitals. Such adjustments can be criticized for not adequately reflecting the more complex case-mix that may characterize teaching hospitals, even when only very high-variation DRGs are analyzed. These very high-variation DRGs can be considered individually to see the extent to which the cases least susceptible to physician discretion come to the teaching hospitals. Finally, as done with regard to the PHS measure, additional variables can be incorporated as controls.

Any new measure benefits from extensive testing. As is noted by Roos and others (51), the PHS measure can be improved. Instrument development should focus on the following issues:

—accuracy of assigning individuals to physicians
—goodness of case-mix adjustment
—goodness of adjustment for characteristics of physicians and hospitals
—robustness of the measures
—consistency of utilization patterns

REFERENCES

1. Hulka, B.S., and Wheat, J.R. Patterns of utilization: The patient perspective. *Med Care* 23:438–60 (1985).
2. Gross, M.J., and Schwenger, C.W. *Health Care Costs for the Elderly in Ontario, 1976–2026*. Ontario Economic Council, Occasional Paper 2 (1981).
3. Wennberg, J.E. On patient need, equity, supplier-induced demand, and the need to assess the outcome of common medical practices. *Med Care* 23:512–20 (1985).
4. Wennberg, J.E., and Fowler, F.J. A test of consumer contribution to small-area variations in health care delivery. *J Maine Med Assoc* 68:275–79 (1977).
5. Roos, N.P., and Roos, L.L. High and low surgical rates: Risk factors for area residents. *Am J Pub Hlth* 71:591–600 (1981).
6. Wennberg, J.E. Dealing with medical practice variations: A proposal for action. *Health Affairs* 3:6–32 (1984).
7. McPherson, K., Hovind, O.B., Clifford, P., and Wennberg, J.E. Small-area variations in the use of common surgical procedures: An international comparison of New England, England, and Norway. *N Eng J Med* 307:1310–14 (1982).
8. Roos, L.L. Supply, workload, and utilization: A population-based analysis of surgery. *Am J Pub Hlth* 73:414–21 (1983).
9. Vayda, E., and Mindell, W.R. Variations in operative rates: What do they mean? *Surg Clin N Amer* 62:627–39 (1982).
10. Smith, C.T. High expectations versus limited resources. *Health Affairs* 5:86–90 (1986).
11. Wennberg, J.E., McPherson, K., and Caper, P. Will payment based on diagnosis-related groups control hospital costs? *N Eng J Med* 311:295–300 (1984).
12. Eisenberg, J.M. *Doctors' Decisions and the Cost of Medical Care*. Ann Arbor, Michigan: Health Administration Press Perspectives (1986).
13. Barer, M.L., and Evans, R.G. Riding north on a south-bound horse? Expenditures, prices, utilization, and incomes in the Canadian health care system. *In:* Evans, R.G., and Stoddard, G.L., eds., *Medicare at Maturity: Lessons from the Past, Challenges for the Future*. Calgary: University of Calgary Press (1986).
14. Roos, N.P., Shapiro, E., and Havens, B.J. Aging with limited resources: What should we really be worried about? *In:* Economic Council of Canada, *Aging with Limited Health Resources*. Ottawa: Canadian Government Publishing Centre (1987).
15. Wolfe, B.L., and Detmer, D.E. The economics of surgical signatures. *Hospital Medical Staff*, October 2–8 (1984).
16. Lohr, K.N., Brook, R.H., Kamberg, C.J., et al. Use of medical care in the Rand Health Insurance Experiment: Diagnosis- and service-specific analyses in a randomized controlled trial. *Med Care (Suppl.)* 24:1–87 (1986).

17. Knickman, J.R., and Foltz, A.M. Regional differences in hospital utilization. How much can be traced to population differences? *Med Care* 22:971–86 (1984).
18. Bloor, M.J., Venters, G.A., and Samphier, M.L. Geographical variation in the incidence of operations on the tonsils and adenoids: An epidemiological and sociological investigation. Parts 1 and 2. *J Laryn Otol* 92:791–801, 883–95 (1979).
19. Rosenblatt, R.A., and Moscovice, I.S. The physician as gatekeeper: Determinants of physicians' hospitalization rates. *Med Care* 22:150–59 (1984).
20. Eisenberg, J.M. Physician utilization: The state of research about physicians' practice patterns. *Med Care* 23:461–83 (1985).
21. Connell, F.A., Blide, L.A., and Hanken, M.A. Clinical correlates of small-area variations in population-based admission rates for diabetes. *Med Care* 22:939–49 (1984).
22. Roos, N.P., Henteleff, P.D., and Roos, L.L. A new audit procedure applied to an old question: Is the frequency of T & A justified? *Med Care* 15:1–18 (1977).
23. Griffith, J.R., et al. Measuring community hospital services in Michigan. *Hlth Serv Res* 16:136–73 (1981).
24. Moore, F.D. Small-area variations studies: Illuminating or misleading? *Health Affairs* 4:96–101 (1985).
25. Schroeder, S.A. Reviews: A medical educator. *Health Affairs* 3:55–62 (1984).
26. Sammons, J.H. Reviews: Organized medicine. *Health Affairs* 3:33–62 (1984).
27. McMahon, L.F., and Newbold, R. Variation in resource use within diagnosis-related groups: The effect of severity of illness and physician practice. *Med Care* 24:388–97 (1986).
28. Wilensky, G.R., and Rossiter, L.F. Patient self-selection in HMOs. *Health Affairs* 5:66–80 (1986).
29. Roch, D.J., Evans, R.G., and Pascoe, D.W. *Manitoba and Medicare—1971 to the Present.* Department of Research Manitoba Health (1985).
30. McCarthy, E.G., and Finkel, M.L. Second-opinion elective programs: Outcome status over time. *Med Care* 16:984–91 (1978).
31. Park, R.E., Fink, A., Brook, R.H., et al. Physician ratings of appropriate indications for six medical and surgical procedures. *Am J Pub Hlth* 76:766–72 (1986).
32. Rutkow, I.M., Gittelsohn, A.M., and Zuideman, G.D. Surgical decision making: The reliability of clinical judgment. *Ann Surg* 190:409–19 (1979).
33. Kissick, W.L., Engstrom, P.F., Soper, K.A., et al. Comparison of internist and oncologist evaluations of cancer patients' need for hospitalization. *Med Care* 22:447–52 (1984).
34. Hemenway, D., and Fallon, D. Testing for physician-induced demand with hypothetical cases. *Med Care* 23:344–49 (1985).
35. Vayda, E., Mindell, W.R., Mueller, C.B., et al. Measuring surgical decision-making with hypothetical cases. *Can Med Assoc J* 127:287–90 (1982).

36. Vayda, E., Mindell, W.R., and Rutkow, I.M. A decade of surgery in Canada, England and Wales, and the United States. *Arch Surg* 117:846–53 (1982).
37. Jensen, J., and Jackson, B. Consumers prefer same-day surgery to inpatient care for minor procedures. *Mod Hlthcare* 15:76–78 (1985).
38. Muller, C. Outpatient surgery: Are we satisfied? *Am J Pub Hlth* 76:1086–87 (1986).
39. Lagoe, R.J., and Milliren, J.W. A community-based analysis of ambulatory utilization. *Am J Pub Hlth* 76:150–53 (1986).
40. Detmer, D.E., and Buchanan-Davidson, D.J. Ambulatory surgery. *Surg Clin N Amer* 62:685–704 (1982).
41. Wennberg, J.E., Barnes, B.A., and Zubkoff, M. Professional uncertainty and the problem of supplier-induced demand. *Soc Sci and Med* 16:811–24 (1982).
42. Sackett, D.L. Clinical disagreement. 1: How often it occurs and why? *Can Med Assoc J* 123:499–504 (1980).
43. Roos, L.L., Nicol, J.P., Johnson, C., and Roos, N.P. Using administrative data banks for research and evaluation: A case study. *Eval Q* 3:236–55 (1979).
44. Roos, L.L., Roos, N.P., Cageorge, S.M., and Nicol, J.P. How good are the data? Reliability of one health care data bank. *Med Care* 20: 266–76 (1982).
45. Demlo, L.K., Campbell, P.M., and Brown, S.S. Reliability of information abstracted from patients' medical records. *Med Care* 16:995–1005 (1978).
46. Demlo, L.K., and Campbell, P.M. Improving hospital discharge data: Lessons from the National Hospital Discharge Survey. *Med Care* 19:1030–40 (1981).
47. Fetter, R.B., Youngsoo, S., Freeman, J.L., et al. Case-mix definition by diagnosis-related groups. *Med Care* 18:1–53 (1980).
48. Fetter, R.B., and Freeman, J.L. Diagnosis-related groups: Product line management within hospitals. *Academy of Management Review* 11:41–54 (1986).
49. Roos, N.P., Wennberg, J.E., and McPherson, K. Using DRGs for studying variations in hospital admission patterns. *Health Care Fin Rev* (forthcoming 1988).
50. Carter, G.M., and Ginsberg, P.B. The Medicare case-mix index increase: Medical practice changes, aging, and DRG creep. Santa Monica, Calif.: Rand Corporation 1985.
51. Roos, N.P., Flowerdew, G., Wajda, A., and Tate, R.B. Variations in physicians' hospitalization practices: A population-based study in Manitoba, Canada. *Am J Pub Hlth* 76:45–51 (1986).
52. Roos, L.L., Cageorge, S.M., Austen, E., and Lohr, K.N. Using computers to identify complications after surgery. *Am J Pub Hlth* 75:1288–95 (1985).
53. Roos, L.L., Cageorge, S.M., Roos, N.P., and Danzinger, R.G. Centralization, certification, and monitoring: Readmissions and complications after surgery. *Med Care* 24:1044–66 (1986).
54. Scitovsky, A.A. The high cost of dying: What do the data show? *Millbank Mem Fund Q* 62:591–608 (1984).

55. Lubitz, J., and Prihoda, R. The use and costs of Medicare services in the last two years of life. *Health Care Fin Rev* 5:117–31 (1984).
56. McCall, N. Utilization and costs of Medicare services by beneficiaries in their last year of life. *Med Care* 22:329–42 (1984).
57. Gillick, M.R., Serrell, N.A., and Gillick, L.S. Adverse consequences of hospitalization in the elderly. *Soc Sci and Med* 16:1033–38 (1982).
58. Dyck, F.J., Murphy, F.A., Murphy, J.K., et al. Effect of surveillance on the number of hysterectomies in the province of Saskatchewan. *N Eng J Med* 296:1326–28 (1977).
59. Mossey, J.M., Havens, B., Roos, N.P., and Shapiro, E. The Manitoba longitudinal study on aging: Description and methods. *Gerontologist* 21:551–58 (1981).
60. Shapiro, E., and Roos, N.P. The Manitoba longitudinal study on aging: Preliminary findings on health care utilization by the elderly. *Med Care* 19:644–57 (1981).
61. Mossey, J.M., and Roos, L.L. Using claims to measure health status: The illness scale. *J Chron Dis* 40:41–49 (1987).
62. Wennberg, J.E., Roos, N.P., Sola, L., et al. Use of claims-data systems to evaluate health care outcomes: Mortality and reoperation following prostatectomy. *JAMA* 257:933–36 (1987).
63. Barer, M.L., Evans, R.G., Hertzman, C., and Lomas, J. Aging and health care utilization: New evidence on old fallacies. *Soc Sci and Med* 24:851–62 (1987).
64. Wennberg, J.E. Factors governing utilization of hospital services. *Hosp Prac* 14:115–27 (1979).
65. Paradise, J.L., Bluestone, C.D., Bachman, R.Z., et al. History of recurrent sore throat as an indication of tonsillectomy. *N Eng J Med* 298:409–13 (1978).
66. Roos, L.L., and Payne, H. Health care evaluation in a government agency: Goals, organization, and software. *Can J Prog Eval* 2:9–15 (1987).
67. Lomas, J., Stoddart, G.L., and Barer, M.L. Supply projections as planning: A critical review of forecasting net physician requirements in Canada. *Soc Sci and Med* 20:411–24 (1985).

7 Surgery and the Changing System of Health Care Delivery

Dan Ermann, M.B.A., M.P.H.

As the makers of public policy and the private payers of health services have become more concerned with the rising cost of delivering health care, there has been a concomitant increase in attention to patterns of surgical care. This interest in surgery has been spurred by both the high societal cost of surgery and questions related to the performance of unnecessary surgery. Hospital inpatient care is the most expensive component of health care delivery. In 1983, 45 percent of inpatient hospital discharges were related to surgery. (1)

The health care delivery system has undergone unprecedented change during the 1980s, affecting health services in general and the practice of surgery in particular. We have witnessed the introduction and rapid growth of multihospital systems, freestanding ambulatory care facilities, health maintenance organizations, and preferred provider organizations. In addition to these organizational changes, technological improvements in diagnostic devices, the development of rapidly acting anesthetics, and advances in the development of microsurgery equipment have taken place. These innovations have made possible the introduction of new medical and surgical procedures as well as improving established modalities of providing care. Surplus hospital capacity and an increasing number of physicians are also resulting in shifts in the delivery of health services. Although hospitals and physicians have competed for years with special amenities and other attractions, they have only recently begun to exhibit competitive prices.

The views expressed in this chapter are those of the author; no official endorsement by the National Center for Health Services Research and Health Care Technology Assessment is intended or should be inferred. The author wishes to thank the following individuals for their helpful comments on earlier drafts of this chapter; which was completed in May 1986: Phyllis Ermann, Ernest Feigenbaum, Jon Gabel, Pam Polister, Ira Raskin, and Larry Rose.

There has been a marked expansion in utilization review activities. Although it has existed for decades, new competitive pressures and improved data and analytical techniques have heightened the interest in, and expectations of, utilization review. Simultaneously, changes in public reimbursement policies (e.g., Medicare) and private insurance coverage place greater financial risk on both the provider and recipient of health services.

This chapter examines the impact of the changing delivery of health care on the provision of surgical services. I address the following questions: What has been the effect of organizational changes on the provision of surgery? How have reimbursement changes, the introduction of greater financial risk for the provider and consumer, and utilization control mechanisms affected surgical services? I conclude with a discussion of the policy implications of system changes and the need for additional research.

ORGANIZATIONAL CHANGES

Ambulatory Surgery Units

The most dramatic transformation in the delivery of surgical care has been the proliferation of ambulatory surgery, defined as the "provision of surgical services that require anesthesia or a period of postoperative observation, or both, to patients whose admission for an overnight stay is not anticipated as being medically necessary" (2). Ambulatory surgery is also referred to as "day surgery," "in-and-out surgery," and "outpatient surgery." Although these different nomenclatures add to the difficulty in identifying and counting ambulatory surgery units and procedures, they all refer to the same basic concept.

Most surgery prior to 1900 was performed in the home. High infection rates in hospitals, and the view of the hospital as a house of death, discouraged the performance of surgery in those primitive facilities. In addition, both patient and physician feared losing the privacy and control available at home. After Lister's work on antisepsis in 1867 and the introduction of X-rays in 1895, more complex surgery began to be performed in hospitals, which offered a safer, technologically superior setting than the home (3). The first outpatient surgery clinic in the United States was established in Sioux City, Iowa, in 1918 (4). However, for years concerns over quality, lack of physician support and insurance coverage, and a limited choice of effective anesthetics restrained the growth of ambulatory surgery (5).

In 1961 the Kaiser-Permanente Medical Care Program in Portland,

Oregon, treated 10 percent of its surgical patients on a "do-not-admit" ambulatory basis. The first freestanding ambulatory surgery center (FASC) in the United States opened in Providence, Rhode Island, in 1968, but failed owing to a lack of support by providers and the decision by Blue Cross not to reimburse patients for procedures performed at the center. The first successful FASC was opened in 1970 in Phoenix, Arizona, under the name Surgicenter and is still in operation (4).

Experts have estimated that between 20 and 40 percent (6) of the approximately 21 million surgical procedures performed annually could be performed in ambulatory settings (7). As a result of recent developments in laser technology, fiber optics, and anesthesia techniques, these estimates are being revised upward and approach 60 percent (8). The potential for ambulatory surgery varies by specialty, with estimates as high as 52–73 percent for urology (9). In 1982, only 20 percent of all surgery was performed on an ambulatory basis, and most of that was in hospital settings (8). Some experts predict that by 1990 we will achieve the earlier goal of 40 percent ambulatory surgery (10).

The choice of ambulatory versus inpatient surgery is influenced by both the patient and the provider and by characteristics of the health care system. Factors of importance are the patient's physical condition and the type of surgery needed, the relative out-of-pocket cost of each alternative setting determined by insurance reimbursement policies, and the patient's personal preferences. However, provider preferences play a dominant role in selection. These may be influenced by financial considerations, concerns about the quality of care, and opportunity costs such as scheduling delays. It has been shown that physicians' practice patterns explain much of the variation in surgical procedure rates. These different practice styles may also influence a physician's choice of setting for delivering care (11–12).

While it is clear that a significant amount of surgery can be performed on an ambulatory basis, the exact amount is difficult if not impossible to ascertain. This uncertainty in part results from the lack of an accepted utilization rate for surgery (by procedure and patient characteristics). As Wennberg and Gittelsohn demonstrated, using small-area analyses, surgery rates vary from area to area without apparent relationship to population needs (12). They hypothesize that differences are caused by variations in the number of practitioners competing for patients and by differences in providers' practice styles. In January 1976, the Subcommittee on Oversight and Investigations of the House Commerce Committee reported that an estimated 2.4 million unnecessary surgeries were performed in 1974 at a loss of 11,900 lives and about $4 billion (13). Therefore, although we can estimate the percentage of surgery that can be performed on an ambulatory basis, we do not know the "correct" total amount of surgery that should be performed. This information would be very helpful in determining the optimal system configuration of ambulatory surgery care units.

Ambulatory surgery facilitities fall into three main categories: (1) an ambulatory surgical unit located within a hospital but integrated with inpatient surgery, (2) a physically and financially autonomous ambulatory surgical unit found within a hospital, and (3) a freestanding ambulatory surgical facility (14). The growth rates of these distinct entities is dissimilar, as is their impact on cost of care. In addition to these arrangements, ambulatory surgery is also performed in physicians' offices, hospital outpatient departments, walk-in clinics, hospital emergency rooms, and independent facilities that perform elective abortions on an outpatient basis (4).

In 1980, 75 percent of nonfederal hospitals in the 134 largest standard metropolitan statistical areas (SMSAs) offered ambulatory surgery services. Seventy percent of all nonfederal hospitals offered ambulatory surgery. This rate varied from a low of 61 percent in the West South Central region to a high of 80 percent in the Mountain region. However, only 54 percent of all hospitals reporting ambulatory surgery services had the necessary facilities and organizational characteristics to be classified as an organized outpatient surgery program (15). By 1984, it was reported that 80 percent of hospital ambulatory surgery programs were performed in inpatient operating rooms; only 2 percent of the hospitals owned or operated freestanding surgery facilities (8). Larger, newer, and not-for-profit hospitals are more likely to offer ambulatory surgery than smaller, older, and for-profit facilities (16). In addition, hospitals with excess capacity and little competition from other ambulatory surgery units are less likely to establish an ambulatory program (17). Hospital-based ambulatory surgery increased 77 percent between 1979 and 1983, while inpatient surgery fell 7 percent (table 7.1 below) (10). Hospital-based ambulatory surgery dominates, accounting for 74 percent of all such surgery, while 20 percent of these operations are performed in physicians' offices and 6 percent are in freestanding facilities (18).

As with many other changes in the delivery of care, we find regional differences in the growth of freestanding facilities. Most freestanding centers are located in the Eastern and Sun Belt regions (with the major concentrations in California, Texas, Illinois, and Florida). One may speculate that regional differences result from differing levels of provider competition, variations in reimbursement coverage, and dissimilar population demographics, which lead to disparate levels of patient demand. Future growth is expected to occur primarily in the Sun Belt (19).

The primary advantages of hospital-affiliated ambulatory units, both independent and integrated, is their ready access to hospital support in an emergency and their increased capability for monitoring quality. Integrated units have the added advantage that limited capital investment is required to set them up. The disadvantages of integrated units include the lower priority given to ambulatory surgery, which results in scheduling problems when both outpatient and inpatient surgery compete for limited resources; the need for more extensive record-keeping for ambulatory patients; and possible disruption to the inpatient facility. In addition, there may be higher costs assigned to ambulatory surgery as a result of cost-accounting procedures that allocate inpatient overhead costs to the ambulatory surgery unit. The ambulatory surgery unit that is financially independent avoids this last obstacle (20).

Freestanding facilities offer a number of advantages, including lower costs, high quality care for a select group of patients, and a pleasant setting tailored to the needs and desires of ambulatory patients. However, there have been a number of barriers to the growth of freestanding centers. Until recently many states employed certificate-of-need programs to regulate the establishment of FASCs. Most states now are eliminating or curtailing these programs. Third-party payers have traditionally reimbursed inpatient care more fully than outpatient. Reimbursement policies are changing to encourage outpatient surgery (as well as other outpatient care). These facilities require large initial capital outlays, and the venture capital market has only recently become interested in the health sector. Finally, health providers have been hesitant to use new delivery settings. But with the growing supply of physicians, and declining hospital occupancy, providers are now willing and even eager to operate and compete in new settings.

The provider community, once hostile to ambulatory surgery, now accepts it. The American Medical Association endorsed the practice in 1971, and by 1981 the American College of Surgeons had approved the increased use of freestanding surgery centers (11). Health insurers are also contributing to the demand for ambulatory surgery. For example, Blue Cross and Blue Shield of Northeastern Ohio has a list of one hundred operations that must be performed as ambulatory procedures unless the patient has contravening complications. This is not atypical, although the list of surgical procedures that can, or must, be performed on an ambulatory basis varies by insurer and from state to state (11). In addition, many payers are now providing more complete insurance coverage for ambulatory surgery than for inpatient care, for example, through lower copayments for ambulatory surgery (21).

Much of the impetus for encouraging ambulatory surgery has come from employers. Recent surveys have shown that American business views ambulatory surgery as a key cost-containment strategy (22). In addition, surveys indicate that approximately 80 percent of the public prefers ambulatory care to inpatient care for minor procedures (23).

Between 1982 and 1983, freestanding ambulatory surgical centers increased in number by 186 percent and other ambulatory surgery centers grew by 283 percent (24). By March 1984, there were 303 freestanding ambulatory surgery centers; 243 in operation and 60 under development. Of these, 63 percent were independently owned, 27 percent were part of corporate surgicenter chains, and only 10 percent were affiliated with a hospital (25). The number of FASCs would be larger if specialty facilities such as opthalmic centers (of which there are approximately 600 in number) were counted (26). The lack of a single accrediting or licensing body, and a multitude of definitions, contribute to the paucity of reliable data.

The primary factor encouraging the growth of ambulatory surgery is the cost-savings potential of this approach. There are numerous reports of savings attributable to ambulatory surgery (21). All of these studies are noteworthy, but I have identified five that specifically compare the costs of ambulatory surgery and inpatient surgery (table 7.1) (27–31). For the most part, these studies compare one facility in each category (i.e., inpatient or FASC) and use charges as the measure of cost. All of them conclude that freestanding centers are least expensive, hospital-based ambulatory surgery next, and inpatient care most costly.

There are two methodologic flaws inherent in these studies. First, they fail to adjust for severity of case mix. Therefore, although the comparisons are for similar procedures, we don't know if patients in certain settings (i.e., inpatient) are sicker or have more medical problems. Second, the use of charges is not a precise measure of costs. It does not adjust for different accounting methods, nor for the possibility of cross-subsidization from profitable to financially weak services.

Savings from ambulatory surgery are primarily due to the elimination of overnight stays before and after surgery, in addition to some savings associated with the surgery. Based on a study of over 60,000 patients at one freestanding surgery center from 1970 to 1980, substantial savings were attributable to the limitation of routine tests, chest X-rays, and electrocardiograms (32). Ambulatory surgery has been estimated to save one to three days of hospitalization. If 50 to 60 percent of the nation's surgery were performed in an ambulatory setting, we could save approximately 600 million inpatient days per year (33). Savings attributable to this reduced utilization depend on the marginal cost of hospital care and on assumption regarding the disposition of excess capacity. However, it is also possible that the availability of ambulatory

TABLE 7.1. Empirical Studies on the Effects of Freestanding Ambulatory Surgery Centers on the Cost of Care

Author	Study Design	Findings
Wolff and Dunnihoo 1982 (27)	Compared costs per case for curettage and laparoscopy between a FASC, an inpatient surgery unit, and a hospital ambulatory unit. Data are for 1978–81.	Costs per case were least at the FASC, were higher in the ambulatory setting, and inpatient care was most expensive. The FASC had the lowest rate of increase in costs over the four-year period.
Maker 1977 (28)	Compared a FASC (Phoenix Surgicenter), hospital inpatient, and hospital ambulatory surgery units for charges for eleven surgical procedures.	The FASC charges were 42–62% lower than the hospital inpatient costs. FASC charges were 17–45 percent lower than those of hospital-affiliated freestanding units. FASC charges were nearly 12 percent lower than those for a hospital outpatient surgical unit. Hospital-based units had a greater use of lab tests and ancillary services.
Maher 1980 (29)	Comparative study of one hospital-owned FASC with inpatient surgical charges (including average inpatient per diem charges) of a nearby hospital.	Patients spent the least time in hospital-affiliated ambulatory surgical units, more time in hospital outpatient settings, and the longest stays were in inpatient surgery units (FASC units were not included in this analysis). FASC patients spent the least time receiving pre- and postoperative services. Time was converted to dollars using 1975 dollars for a median annual earning for a full-time, year-round, male worker. Thus the most economical unit was the FASC.
Jagger et al. 1978 (30)	Comparison of total operating costs for three comparable surgical procedures performed in FASC and hospital outpatient surgery department.	Slightly lower costs (but not statistically significant) in the FASC than the outpatient unit.
Beazley 1980 (31)	Compared costs per case for D & Cs and breast biopsies performed on inpatient and outpatient basis at one hospital.	Outpatient costs were one-third less for D & C operations and half for breast biopsies.

surgery facilities will result in increased utilization, and possibly in an increase in total surgery costs. No empirical analysis of the effect of ambulatory surgery on total system expenditures has been conducted.

No study has considered the costs associated with any possible extended recuperation period at home when surgery is performed on an ambulatory basis. This should include direct cost of home care, plus lost income for family members who must stay home to care for the patient. In addition, the effect of increased ambulatory surgery on hospitals, already coping with reduced utilization, will be significant. As inpatient demand decreases, and the mix of cases becomes more complex (and costly), hospitals will realize additional cost pressures. One solution being undertaken by many hospitals is to diversify further into ambulatory care services.

The second major issue is that of the quality of care. What type of care do ambulatory units provide? Eight empirical studies examine the impact of ambulatory surgery on the quality of care (27, 28, 32, 34–38). Measures of quality include death rates, complications, and transfers to hospitals. Ambulatory surgical outcomes have been impressive (in terms of the small number of surgical deaths and complications). The studies (see table 7.2) indicate that ambulatory patients have experienced a relatively low rate of complications and transfers to a hospital after surgery. This has been attributed to "careful screening of the patients prior to surgery" (39). In one Chicago ambulatory surgery unit, almost 50 percent of patients were under twenty years old, while only 3 percent were over sixty. In addition, 97 percent were considered in good health, and only 3 percent showed evidence of a serious systemic disease (34). A study by Professional Research Consultants corroborated this. They found that higher income, younger, and better educated persons were more likely to utilize ambulatory surgery facilities (40). Low postsurgical infection rates for ambulatory surgery are also a benefit of avoiding inpatient care. One study reported that 17 percent of pediatric patients admitted for hernia surgery acquired upper respiratory or gastrointestinal tract infection (41) The incidence of such infections can be reduced by up to 70 percent when the operations are done on an ambulatory basis (42).

The Free-Standing Ambulatory Surgery Association reported that the ten most common procedures in thirty-nine responding facilities accounted for 72 percent of all ambulatory surgical procedures in 1981 (table 7.3) (43). An analysis of these procedures indicates careful selection of cases. Procedures are generally those of short duration (15–90 minutes), associated with minimal bleeding and minor physiologic derangement. They also have a predictably low infection rate (44). The most frequent procedures are performed by gynecologists, ear, nose,

TABLE 7.2. Empirical Studies on the Effects of Freestanding Ambulatory Surgery Centers on Quality of Care

Author	Study Design	Findings
Natof 1980 (34)	Studied 13,433 patients at forty-nine FASCs through the first two postoperative weeks	Identified 106 medical, surgical, and anesthetic complications. No deaths occurred at the FASC. Sixteen patients were transferred to a general hospital.
Maker 1977 (28)	Studied six FASCs.	Found that appropriate screening was used to eliminate any high-risk patients from receiving care at the FASC. Three unscheduled patient transfers occurred in 900 sampled.
Knapp 1981 (35)	Studied 21,000 patients receiving care at a FASC and transfers to a hospital following surgery	Found thirty-two transfers to hospitals after surgery; only three were made by ambulance.
Bruns 1981 (36)	Analyzed all 76,581 procedures reported in 1980.	Found 10,767 complications (14.1 percent). If nausea and vomiting (the most common) are omitted, the complication rate is 5.4 percent. There were 223 patients who required hospitaliation following surgery, and 8 had emergency or life-threatening complications.
Bruns 1982 (37)	Studied the quality of care (in terms of transfers of nearly 500,000 surgical procedures in thirty-six facilities from 1972 to 1980.	There were 233 patient transfers to a hospital; 89 of these were unanticipated, and 8 were emergency transfers. There were no fatalities.
Wolff and Dunihoo 1982 (27)	Studied 5,369 surgical patients receiving care at one FASC in Louisiana between August 1978 and January 1981.	Found three superficial wound infections and two hospital transfers.
Bruns 1982 (38)	Compiled statistics from fourteen responding FASCs regarding complication rates for 33,662 procedures.	Reported 16.1 percent complication rate with 128 major complications. In twelve cases, complications required hospitalization for dire or life-threatening circumstances. There were 153 transfers to hospitals without dire need, and 44 patients were hospitalized after surgery. There was one reported death in 552,895 cases.

(*Continued*)

TABLE 7.2. (Continued)

Author	Study Design	Findings
Dawson and Reed 1980 (32)	Analyzed data on more than 60,000 patients at one FASC from 1970 to 1979.	The most common complications were nausea (30 percent of patients) and emesis (20 percent of patients). The hospital transfer rate was 0.2 percent for all patients and 0.59 percent for patients over sixty-four years old. No patient was transferred as an emergency, most transfers were for bleeding, inadequate pain relief, and further elective operations.

and throat surgeons, orthopedic surgeons, plastic surgeons, and general surgery specialists. Of the ten most common surgical procedures performed in hospitals, six can now be performed in an ambulatory setting on some (but not all) patients (4).

Health Maintenance Organizations,
Preferred Provider Organizations, and Multihospital Systems

Health maintenance organizations (HMOs), preferred provider organizations (PPOs), and multihospital systems have proliferated in recent years and they continue to expand. As they multiply and mature, their impact on the total health care delivery system also intensifies.

An HMO is an organization that delivers a stated range of health services to a defined enrolled population for a fixed monthly or annual premium. Typically, physicians working for the HMO (either directly employed or under contract) receive financial incentives for controlling costs through conservative use of health services and facilities. The first HMO, the Ross-Loos Health Plan, was organized in 1929. It is only in recent years, however, that HMOs have seen growth. HMO enrollment grew 21 percent from 1983 to 1984, and 25 percent from 1984 to 1985 (45). Currently, more than 20 million Americans belong to an HMO (46). Much of this growth has been spurred by the strong belief that HMOs provide high-quality care at lower cost than the fee-for-service arrangement.

In 1984, the Rand Health Insurance Experiment reported that HMOs, when compared to fee-for-service practice in a randomized controlled experiment, delivered health care with 40 percent fewer hospital admissions and a 75 percent cost reduction. The researchers concluded that the style of medicine practiced in HMOs is less hospital intensive

TABLE 7.3 Top FASC Procedures for 1981

Name	Number	Percentage of Total
Dilation and curettage	14,148	14.9
Laparoscopy	10,849	11.5
Orthopedic procedures	9,855	10.4
Myringotomy	9,081	9.6
Excision of skin lesion	8,610	8.6
Arthroscopy	4,124	4.3
Tonsillectomy/adenoidectomy	3,716	3.9
Dental procedures	3,267	3.4
Plastic surgery	3,106	3.2
Cystocopy	1,924	2.0
Total	68,230	72.2

Source: Reference 37.

(47). A review of the research literature found that quality of surgical care in established HMOs is comparable or better than in traditional fee-for-service settings (48). In addition, patients in the fee-for-service setting are more likely to have unnecessary surgery. HMO patients, on the other hand, are less likely to undergo elective surgery. The researchers concluded that large group structures, organized group networks, and third-party cost-reducing incentives contribute to the HMO success in controlling surgery rates. HMOs emphasize ambulatory, nonspecialist care. This may have widespread implications as HMOs sign contracts with more hospitals to provide care to their enrollees. It has not been determined whether contracting hospitals will modify their delivery approach as a consequence, thereby providing more ambulatory surgery to non-HMO patients, or whether they will attempt to compensate for reduced HMO utilization by increasing non-HMO inpatient use.

A more recent entrant into the health field is the preferred provider organization. A PPO may be an organization, a delivery system, or an arrangement between providers and third-party payers. The providers agree to provide service to a specific group of patients, usually on a discounted fee-for-service basis. Subscribers are usually members of an employer group and are given financial incentives to use the preferred providers, but they retain the right to choose other providers. Providers are promised an increased pool of patients and more rapid payment of claims. The third-party payer or self-insured employer, rather than the provider, generally assumes the financial risk for unanticipated utilization. The growth of PPOs has been phenomenal. In December 1984, it was estimated that about 1.3 million persons were eligible to use a PPO (49). By July 1985, approximately 6 million persons were eligible (50). In the winter of 1986, the number of persons eligible probably approached 10 to 12 million.

It now appears that utilization review is the major means for controlling costs in PPOs. A survey conducted in the spring of 1985 found that virtually all PPOs used at least one form of utilization review. These review mechanisms, aimed primarily at controlling hospital inpatient care, are becoming more sophisticated and purportedly more effective. Furthermore, utilization review programs should begin to identify "unnecessary" inpatient surgery, thus reducing inpatient care. Forty-three percent of surveyed PPOs reported that they were operating mandatory second-opinion surgery programs. Utilization review of ambulatory care is still in the developmental stage. There is as yet limited ability to identify or monitor the need for ambulatory surgery procedures. Although no empirical evidence exists documenting the effect of PPOs on ambulatory surgery, it is reasonable to assume that ambulatory surgery will become the preferred treatment setting for PPO patients. The 1985 survey found that 52 percent of PPOs had signed contracts with ambulatory centers (50).

The third major shift in the health care delivery system has been the increasing prominence of the multihospital system, two or more hospitals that are owned, managed, or leased by a single organization. In 1982, one of every three U.S. hospitals, comprising nearly 36 percent of the nation's hospital beds, belonged to a multihospital system (51). Since 1982, the growth of multihospital systems has continued. Why would one expect multihospital systems to affect ambulatory surgery? Two reasons become apparent. First, multihospital systems have historically been successful at modifying their strategies and behavior in order to compete in a changing environment. With the introduction of the Medicare prospective payment system (DRGs), and increased competition in the health sector, hospitals are encouraged to become more efficient and innovative in their delivery of services. Hospital-owned ambulatory surgery units allow the hospital to compete and retain its market share while better utilizing the inpatient facility for acute-care patients. Second, these organizations have both the organizational will and the resources to diversify into outpatient care. Their purported advantage in capital acquisition and improved information systems should facilitate their expansion in the outpatient care sector.

One research effort surveyed multihospital systems and compared their mix of out-of-hospital services to a group of comparable independent hospitals (52). Based on preliminary analysis, no statistically significant difference existed between the percentage of system hospitals (78.4 percent of 577 hospitals) and that of independent hospitals (81.7 percent of 300 hospitals) that offered ambulatory surgery. Both groups offered ambulatory surgery to a significant degree. It is interesting to note that both investor-owned and not-for-profit systems perceived a

TABLE 7.4. Perceived Market Growth Potential (Moderate or High Growth)

	Inpatient Surgery	Ambulatory Surgery
Investor-owned systems	41.8%	74.9%
Not-for-profit	25.8%	70.3%

much greater growth potential for ambulatory surgery than for inpatient surgery (see table 7.4).

UTILIZATION REVIEW AND REIMBURSEMENT CHANGES

Utilization Review Activities

To date, most utilization review programs have targeted hospital inpatient care, with only limited interest in ambulatory care. This has occurred because of the large financial resources consumed by the hospital sector and the dearth of reliable data on out-of-hospital care. There are also a more manageable number of hospitals to deal with compared with the multitude of physicians' offices. While the primary goal of utilization review programs is cost containment, they also may institutionalize a system for monitoring the quality of services provided.

Hospital utilization review primarily takes two forms: certification of prospective admissions and concurrent review of hospitalized patients. Preadmission certification is used to screen-out unnecessary hospital admissions, often referring the patient to an alternate setting. Concurrent review is used to monitor the hospitalization, assuring that a patient will not remain in the facility longer than may be medically necessary. Findings indicate that concurrent review has only a negligible overall impact on the length of hospital stay, and hence on cost-containment goals. However, preadmission certification could contribute significantly to the containment of hospital utilization (53). Preadmission screening assures that the planned elective or nonemergency hospitalization is medically necessary and is provided in an appropriate setting. If performed properly, preadmission review will channel patients for minor surgery to alternative settings (e.g., hospital ambulatory or freestanding surgery facilities) when these are available.

Second-opinion surgery programs are designed to prevent unnecessary surgery by encouraging or requiring patients to seek advice from a second physician before deciding whether to undergo surgery. Second-opinion programs have existed since the early 1970s. Researchers have attempted to evaluate these programs in terms of their effect on surgical rates and associated costs. They have been less successful in estimating the "sentinel" effect, that is, the degree to which a program's existence prompts physicians to become more conservative in making initial recommendations for surgery.

Eight studies I examined estimate the effects of mandatory second-opinion programs on surgery rates. Estimates of reduction in the surgery rates among mandatory program participants range from 3 to 23 percent. However, these studies have not controlled for other factors affecting surgery rates, and therefore the studies may have overestimated program effects (54). For voluntary programs, a reduction among program participants of 12 percent was found, corresponding to a reduction of 0.3 percent in the covered population (55). This discrepancy resulted from the relatively small number of people who use the program. Another study of a voluntary second-opinion surgery program found that it induced more surgery than it prevented. More patients, who would not otherwise have had surgery, underwent an operation after agreement between the two surgeons than the number of patients discouraged from surgery because of differing opinions (56).

In sum, only mandatory programs appear to result in substantial savings, with no apparent direct effects on the health outcomes of participants. There is an absence of information on the indirect influence of these programs on patient health as related to, for example, changes in physician behavior due to the sentinel effect.

Reimbursement Changes

Government and private insurers have modified their insurance coverage to encourage the use of ambulatory surgery units. The Omnibus Budget Reconciliation Act of 1980 (P.L. 96-499) "endorsed the concept of ambulatory surgery and sought to eliminate the pro-hospital bias of the original Medicare legislation." As a result, ambulatory surgery facilities were approved for Medicare reimbursement (19). Both the Medicare program and private insurers have developed lists of surgical procedures that either may, or must, be performed on an outpatient basis. In 1982, Medicare published a list of one hundred procedures that were reimbursable only if they were performed in an ambulatory surgery center (ASC), that is, a center accredited by Medicare. This list is periodically updated. Medicare also encourages physicians to use ASCs by reimbursing them 100 percent if they accept assignment of an ASC. If physicians use a hospital for surgery and accept assignment, they collect 80 percent of the allowable charge from Medicare and must collect the remainder from the patient (57).

Some employers, such as Mobil Oil (New York), have introduced stronger incentives for employees to use ambulatory surgery by requiring a deductible and copayment for inpatient surgery while reimbursing outpatient surgery in full (58). Maryland Blue Cross, on the other hand, introduced a plan that will not pay at all for some procedures on an inpatient basis unless need can be demonstrated (4). A study by Hewitt Associates indicates that 96 percent of employer-sponsored policies covered ambulatory surgery in 1984, compared to only 35 percent coverage in 1974 (59).

Only a few studies examine the effect of different reimbursement methods on the surgeon's practice style. One such study found marked differences. For example, salaried surgeons performed laboratory tests and radiographic procedures more frequently and less selectively than did their colleagues reimbursed in other arrangements, without any corresponding improvement in outcome (60). The researchers also found some differences in the number of surgical procedures by payment mechanism (e.g., salaried surgeons performed fewer operations than either prepaid or fee-for-service physicians). They concluded that "while oversupply undoubtedly explains the low workload of surgeons in private practice, the method of remuneration may well account for the lower operative load of salaried surgeons."

This chapter does not delve into the complex issue of reimbursement and the influence of various insurance programs on surgical procedure rates and expenditures. Suffice it to say that there is evidence that the payment method affects the practice of medicine in terms of where providers offer care and the quantity and cost of that care.

DISCUSSION

Changes in the organization and reimbursement of health services have contributed to major shifts in the delivery of surgical services. However, the lack of a comprehensive data set and the recency of such changes make this a very difficult issue to study.

The pressures of cost containment, together with concerns over the delivery of unnecessary surgery, will not abate in the near future. Innovative organizational forms, such as PPOs, HMOs, and multihospital systems, will attempt to compete by controlling expensive inpatient care and substituting less costly outpatient care. It is clear that ambulatory surgery, both in hospitals and in freestanding facilities, is growing in importance and acceptance and will continue to spread. Ambulatory surgery is less expensive than inpatient surgery and of high quality for a select population of otherwise healthy patients. Increased sophistication in the development of data sets and analytical techniques (e.g., by utilization review programs) will further spur the movement toward more efficient health service delivery. This implies that hospital inpatient care should be considered as the treatment modality of last resort. Patients will only be treated on an inpatient basis when other less costly alternatives are either unavailable or medically unsuitable.

It is impossible at this time to predict who will reap the benefits of system changes, or who will pay. Insurers and payers will probably benefit with reduced costs and lower utilization of expensive services. Providers (hospitals, physicians, and freestanding facilities) have the opportunity to compete for the first time on the basis of cost. The successful providers will be those who can operate efficiently, while maintaining a desired service of high quality. The unsuccessful providers may face a decline in their practice. Patients can gain through lower health costs and the ability to choose among various providers who offer different "products." However, care delivered must be closely monitored to insure that in the rush to control costs we maintain a system delivering high-quality care. This is especially important as the aged segment of the population increases, with persons aged eighty-three and over constituting the most rapidly growing portion of the population (61).

CONCLUSION

More research is needed on the provision of surgical services. We must evaluate the implications of delivery changes on both the cost and the quality of care. This may only be done using large data sets that capture the occurrence of infrequent events, as well as smaller case studies to examine individual, or unique, approaches before they are in widespread use. While ongoing data collection and analysis systems (such as various hospital discharge programs) have an appeal, there is also a need for one-time studies to examine discrete issues.

REFERENCES

1. National Center for Health Statistics, *Utilization of Short-stay Hospitals: Annual Summary for the U.S., 1983*. Vital and Health Statistics, U.S. Dept. of Health and Human Services (1985).
2. Barron, E., and Noble, J. Ambulatory surgery offers quality savings. *Hospitals* 54:74–76 (1980).
3. Starr, P. *The Social Transformation of American Medicine*. New York: Basic Books (1982).

4. Valentine, W., and Palmer, B. *Ambulatory Surgery Services Methodological Note No. 5.* Office of Health Planning, U.S. Public Health Service, Dept. of Health and Human Services (1984).
5. Natof, H. Outpatient surgery: An alternative. *AORN Journal* 29:659–62 (1979).
6. Davis, J., and Detmer, D. The ambulatory surgical unit. *Ann Surg* 175:856 (1985).
7. *Hospital Statistics.* Chicago: American Hospital Association (1985).
8. Olson, L. Providers preparing for major battle over market for outpatient surgery. *Modern Hlthcare* 14:82–92 (1984).
9. Wagner, D. The surgical ambulatory care unit. *In:* Wolcott, M., ed., *Ferguson's Surgery of the Ambulatory Patient.* Philadelphia: Lippincott (1974).
10. Outpatient surgery up 77 percent: Data. *Hospitals* 59:54 (1985).
11. Wennberg, J. E., and Gittelsohn, A. M. Small-area variations in health care delivery. *Science* 182:1102 (1973).
12. Wennberg, J. E., and Gittelsohn, A. M. Health care delivery in Maine. 1: Patterns of use of common surgical procedures. *J. Maine Med Assoc* 66:123 (1975).
13. *A Mandatory Second Surgical Opinion Would Prove Beneficial to the Medicaid and Medicare Programs.* Office of Inspector General, Dept. of Health and Human Services (1983).
14. Edelist, G., and Urbach, G. Organization of the outpatient surgical facility. *J Can Anesth Soc* 27:4 (1980).
15. Burns, L., and Ferber, M. *Profile on Ambulatory Surgery Program in United States Hospitals.* Chicago: American Hospital Association (1981).
16. Burns, L., and Ferber, M. Survey indicates extensive ambulatory surgery by hospitals. *Hospitals* 55:69 (1981).
17. Burns, L. Will multi-institutional systems serve as change agents to improve the management of ambulatory care? *J Ambulatory Care Mgmt* 8:1–17 (1985).
18. Inguanzo, J., and Marju, M. What's the market for outpatient surgery? *Hospitals* 59:55–57 (1985).
19. Trauner, J., Luft, H., and Robinson, J. *Entrepreneurial Trends in Health Care Delivery: The Development of Retail Dentistry and Freestanding Ambulatory Services.* San Francisco: Institute for Health Policy Studies, University of California (1982).
20. Stetson, P. Hospital-affiliated or freestanding units: Which are best? *AORN Journal* 38:1049–54 (1983).
21. LeRoux, M. Outpatient benefits need right incentive. *Bus Insurance* 17:44 (1983).
22. Gardner, S., Kyzer-Sheeley, B., and Sabatino, B. Big business embraces alternative delivery. *Hospitals* 59:81–82 (1985).
23. Jensen, J., and Jackson, B. Consumers prefer same-day surgery to inpatient care for minor procedures. *Modern Hlthcare* 15:76–78 (1985).
24. Ambulatory surgery: Freestanding centers look beyond growth of early years. *AORN Journal* 42:105–8 (1985).

25. Henderson, J. Surgicenters will mushroom if hospitals don't hobble growth. *Modern Hlthcare* 14:156 (1984).
26. Dean, A. Ambulatory surgery. *Texas Hospital* 38:48–49 (1983).
27. Wolff, J., and Dunnihoo, D. A freestanding ambulatory surgical unit: A success or failure? *Am J Ob Gyn* 143:270 (1982).
28. Maker, J. *Comparative Evaluation of Costs, Quality, and System Effects of Ambulatory Surgery Performed in Alternative Settings—Executive Summary.* Orkand Corp., Dept. of Health, Education, and Welfare (1977).
29. Maher, F. Surgical costs and utilization. *Hospitals* 57:107 (1980).
30. Jaggar, F., et al. Comparative evaluation of the costs, quality, and system effects of ambulatory surgery performed in alternative settings. Paper presented at the 106th annual meeting of the American Public Health Association, Los Angeles, Calif., Oct. 18, 1978.
31. Beazley, W. The trend to outpatient care. 1: In-and-out surgery. *Virginia Med* 107:620–21 (1980).
32. Dawson, B., and Reed, W. Anesthesia for adult surgical outpatients *J Can Anesth Soc* 27:409–11 (1980).
33. Maximizing outpatient surgery could cut 600 million patient days yearly. *Hospitals* 59:61 (1985).
34. Natof, H. Complications associated with ambulatory surgery. *JAMA* 244:92 (1980).
35. Knapp, M. The Wichita Minor Surgery Center: Perspective of the independent freestanding surgery center. *J Ambulatory Care Mgmt* 14:75–84 (1981).
36. Bruns, K. FASA statistics reveal top ten procedures. *Same-Day Surgery* 5:47 (1981).
37. Bruns, K. FASA statistics reveal top ten procedures. *Same-Day Surgery* 6:58 (1982).
38. Bruns, K. *A Statistical Analysis of Freestanding Outpatient Surgical Care Facilities for the Year 1981.* Phoenix: Freestanding Ambulatory Surgical Association (1982).
39. Detmer, D., and Buchanan-Davidson, D. Ambulatory surgery. *Surg Clin N Amer* 62:685–704 (1982).
40. Baldwin, M. Surgery centers pressure HCFA for higher Medicare facility fees. *Mod Hlthcare* 15:63 (1985).
41. Izant, R. Nosocomial infections in a children's hospital. Twenty-seventh Ross Pediatric Research Conference (1958).
42. Otherson, H., and Clatworthy, H. Outpatient herniorraphy for infants. *Am J Dis Child* 116:78–80 (1968).
43. Bruns, K. op cit.
44. Spielman, F. Ambulatory surgery. *Resident and Staff Physician* 29:95 (1983).
45. *HMO Summary, June 1985.* Excelsior, Minn: Interstudy (1985).
46. *HMO Summary, June 1986.* Excelsior, Minn: Interstudy (1986).
47. Stein, J. Industry's new bottom line on health care costs: Is less better? *Hastings Center Report* 15:14–18 (1985).

48. LoGerfo, J. Organizational and financial influences on patterns of care. *Surg Clin N Amer* 62:677–83 (1982).
49. Gabel, J., and Ermann, D. Preferred provider organizations: Performance, problems, and promise. *Health Affairs* 4:24–40 (1985).
50. Rice, T., DeLissovoy, G., Gabel, J., The state of PPOs: Results from a national survey. *Health Affairs* 4:25–40 (1985).
51. Ermann, D., and Gabel, J. Multihospital systems: Issues and empirical findings. *Health Affairs* 3:50–64 (1984).
52. Shortell, S. A study of multi-unit health care systems: Preliminary findings. National Center for Health Services Research and Health Care Technology Assessment, Grant HSO5159 (1986).
53. Baoz, R. Utilization review and containment of hospital utilization: Some implications of providing care in the most appropriate setting. *Med Care* 17:315–30 (1979).
54. Finkel, M. L., McCarthy, E. G., and Ruchlin, H. S. *Second Surgical Opinion Programs: An Analysis of Public Policy Options, Executive Summary.* Health Care Financing Administration, Dept. Health and Human Services. (1985).
55. Poggio, E. *Second Surgical Opinion Programs: An Investigation of Mandatory and Voluntary Alternatives.* Boston: Abt Associates (1981).
56. Schachter, M., Oppenheimer, G., and Cannoodt, T., et al. Evaluation of a surgical second-opinion program. *Quality Rev Bull* 9:11 (1983).
57. Social Security Act. Sec. 1833 i (4)A.
58. U.S. corporations offer incentives to encourage outpatient surgery. *Same-Day Surgery* 5:140–41 (1981).
59. Fruen, M., and Field, M. Ambulatory surgery comes of age. *Business and Health* 2:28 (1985).
60. Wilson, S., and Longmire, W. Does method of surgeon payment affect surgical care? *J. Surg Res* 24:457–68 (1978).
61. Rosenwaike, I. A demographic portrait of the oldest old. *Millbank Mem Fund Q /Health and Society* 63:187–205 (1985).

8 Identifying Hospitals for the Regionalization of Care

Harold S. Luft and Sandra S. Hunt

Routinely collected case-abstract data has proven invaluable for certain types of research that focus on patterns of performance across hospitals. For example, using both measures of morbidity and mortality, a growing body of research indicates that patient outcomes are better in hospital having high volumes of patients with the particular procedure or diagnosis (1–7). This observation has led to the suggestion that policies be developed to encourage patients to be treated in hospitals with high volumes. Not all high-volume hospitals have good outcomes, however, so it will be necessary to identify particular hospitals with better than average performance. Preferred provider organizations and Medicaid programs such as California's have already established contracts with selected hospitals and channel their enrollees toward those hospitals (8). To date, these contracts have not focused on patient outcomes, but quality has been at least a secondary consideration. Even without active efforts to encourage regionalization, case-abstract data can be used to provide consumers with uniform data on hospital outcomes. In fact, the Department of Health and Human Services has released data on hospital-specific outcomes for Medicare patients (9). There have already been some widely discussed instances in which similar data have been used in public settings to criticize specific hospitals and physicians for allegedly poor outcomes (10–13).

While case-abstract data may be adequate for research on outcomes across a large number of hospitals, and while highly significant statistical relationships can be recognized, such data are often inade-

---

An earlier version of this chapter appeared as "Evaluating Hospital Quality through Outcome Statistics" in the *Journal of the American Medical Association* 255:20 (1986) and is used with permission. This research was supported by grant number HS-04329 from the National Center for Health Services Research, Department of Health and Human Services.

We are grateful for comments from Warren Browner, John Bunker, Stephen McPhee, Nancy Ramsay, Susan Sacks, and anonymous reviewers for comments on an earlier draft.

quate for the identification of individual hospitals as having particularly good or poor outcomes. This problem arises from the inherent variability in outcomes across patients with similar diagnoses and treatments, as well as from the relatively low rate of adverse outcomes and small numbers of patients with a particular diagnosis or procedure seen in any one hospital. When hundreds of hospitals and thousands of patients can be included in a study, much of the random variation can be ignored as unexplained "noise". When the focus is just on outcomes in hospital A versus hospital B, however, most of what is seen is probably random variation.

To illustrate this problem, this chapter utilizes case-abstract data for patients undergoing cardiac catheterization in 151 hospitals during 1982. The in-hospital death rate for these patients is approximately 1 percent, a figure about in the middle of the range for procedures and diagnoses. The number of patients undergoing catheterization in particular hospitals is relatively high, reducing the problem of statistical variation and making our presentation of the problems somewhat conservative. It will be shown that while a strong inverse relation exists between mortality for these patients and the volume of similar cases at the hospital, the identification of hospitals with significantly better or worse than average outcomes is quite difficult. The last part of the chapter discusses the application of the approach to categories of patients, with varying volumes and rates of adverse outcomes, and suggests some methods to use similar data to encourage regionalization.

DATA AND METHODS

The data for this study were derived from the Professional Activity Studies (PAS) of the Commission on Professional and Hospital Activities (CPHA), Ann Arbor, Michigan. All 757 hospitals that subscribed to the system for the entire year of 1982 and that were also respondents to the nationwide Survey of Specialized Clinical Services (SSCS) were included. Only 151 of the 757 hospitals in our sample reported having a cardiac catheterization laboratory, and we excluded hospitals reporting catheterizations without having a laboratory. (The 1982 SSCS was sent to all U.S. community hospitals, and responses were received from 3,781, response rate of 66 percent. While small hospitals were somewhat less likely to respond to the SSCS, there were no other significant response biases.)

Patient records were excluded at the outset if data were missing on age, sex, discharge status, or length of stay. To maintain confidentiality, all data were aggregated to the hospital level and identifiers were removed by CPHA. Differences in case mix across hospitals were measured by developing a risk factor matrix based on characteristics known to be associated with differential mortality rates, including age and diagnoses. For cardiac catheterization there were twelve cells (age 35–49, age 50–64, age 65 and over, multiplied by dysrhythmia [ICD9-427], heart failure [ICD9-428], any other single diagnosis, such as renal failure, and any multiple diagnoses). Patients were allocated to the appropriate cells, and cell-specific death rates were then calculated. An expected death rate for each hospital was derived by summing over all cells the national cell-specific death rate times the proportion of patients in the hospital falling into each cell. This indirectly standardized mortality rate, or expected death rate, is what would be anticipated if the hospital achieved outcomes equivalent to the national average within each cell, adjusting for differences in case mix at the hospital level. Expected death rates were calculated for groups of hospitals in an analogous way.

Hospitals were grouped into volume categories according to the number of patients seen in a year within a procedure category. The cutoff levels for each category were determined after examining the distribution of hospitals by volume. Groups were formed with attention to having a reasonable number of patients in each category, and break points were designed to reflect natural patterns in the distribution. Outcome differences were not considered in the formation of groups. For cardiac catheterization, the volume categories are 1–200, 201–400, 401–500, 501–750, and more than 751 patients per year.

Analysis of the relation between volume and outcome uses regression for the evaluation of trends. The binomial distribution is used for the examination of individual hospital outcomes.

Statistical Evidence

Figure 8.1 presents the ratio of actual to expected death for groups of hospitals arranged by volume category. There is a highly significant inverse relation between the number of patients undergoing catheterization in a hospital and the in-hospital mortality rate, adjusting for case mix. The regression of the difference between actual and expected death rates on the log of volume of catheterization patients yields a coefficient of $-.013$, with a p value of .0014. The log form captures the curvilinear relation present in figure 8.1, with substantially higher mortality rates observed at very low volumes. While the causal relationship is still in dispute—that is, does higher volume lead to better outcomes or do better outcomes attract higher volumes—this does not

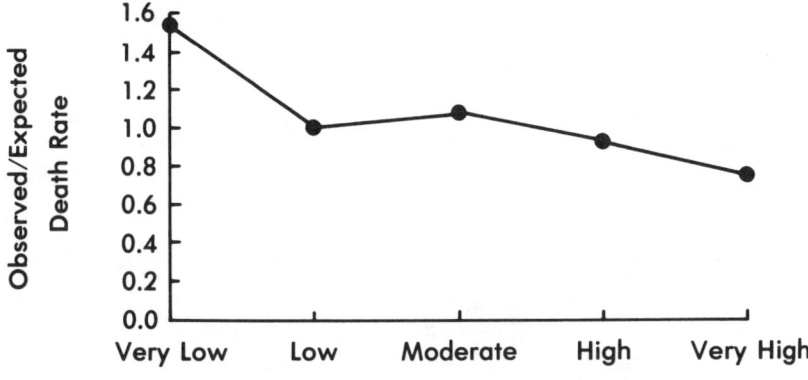

Figure 8.1. Observed/Expected Death Rates for Cardiac Catheterization by Volume Category

affect the issue at hand (1, 2, 5, 14–16). In fact, an inverse relation between volume and outcome for coronary arteriography was first reported by Adams, Fraser, and Abrams in 1973 (17). The question posed in this chapter is whether similar data can be used to identify particular hospitals as having better or worse than average outcomes.

The ratios in figure 8.1 are based upon all deaths in all hospitals within a volume category in the numerator and all patients in the denominator. This reduces the problem of unstable ratios due to small numbers of patients in each hospital that occurs when each hospital is considered separately. Thus one can obtain a more reliable estimate by grouping data. Grouping observations or using techniques such as correlation or regression to abstract from what is effectively random variation or the influence of extraneous factors is reasonable if the focus is on the analysis of a relationship between variables. However, if one is concerned with evaluating the performance of individual hospitals or even groups of hospitals, such methods may suggest more precision than is truly available.

Suppose, then, that one is interested in whether hospitals with very low volumes of patients undergoing cardiac catheterization have outcomes significantly worse than what would be expected given their case mix. Table 8.1 presents the relevant data for hospitals grouped by volume. For the very low-volume hospitals, with 200 or fewer catheterizations per year, the ratio of observed to expected deaths is 1.54, with a 90 percent confidence interval of 1.30 to 1.78. Thus one could be reasonably confident in rejecting the null hypothesis that hospitals with very low catheterization volumes have outcomes similar to the expected

TABLE 8.1. Patient Outcomes for Cardiac Catheterization by Hospital Group

	Very Low	Low	Medium	High	Very High
Volume per year	1–200	200–400	401–500	501–750	750 +
Number of hospitals	31	49	19	27	25
Number of patients	3,484	14,813	8,394	16,122	27,546
Expected deaths	46	190	103	171	283
Observed deaths	70	191	110	157	210
Observed/expected	1.54	1.00	1.07	0.92	0.74
90 percent confidence level					
Lower bound	1.30	0.88	0.90	0.80	0.64
Upper bound	1.78	1.12	1.24	1.05	0.84

rate, given their case mix. At the other extreme, the results for hospitals with very high volumes, more than 750 procedures per year, are significantly better than average (risk ratio = .74, with a 90 percent confidence interval of .64 to .84). Outcomes for the middle groupings are not significantly different from the average, yet it is clear that the relationship between volume and outcome presented in figure 8.1 can be discerned in these data. The difference in perspective is that attention has shifted from the pattern across all hospitals to the performance of specific groups of hospitals.

In table 8.2, individual hospital outcomes are examined. Just as the number of expected deaths can be calculated for groups of hospitals based upon their case mix, analogous estimates of expected deaths can be computed for individual hospitals and then compared with observed deaths. The binomial distribution is used to determine the likelihood that the number of observed deaths came from a distribution with a mean death rate equal to the expected rate in that hospital. In computing these probabilities, we included a continuity correction that smooths the values by averaging the point probabilities associated with N and $N + 1$ bad outcomes.

For individual hospitals, the combination of low probabilities of death and low volumes means that one often expects to observe zero deaths. It is really the case that this provides no useful information about how well the hospital is performing when there are very few patients. In table 8.2 two hospitals met the criteria of extremely low volumes (one and two patients respectively) and zero deaths, and thus were excluded. Both these hospitals reported having catheterization laboratories, although it is possible they began operation only at the end of the year. The next two lowest volume hospitals had thirteen and fifty-two patients, with seven and three deaths, respectively, which was significantly worse than would be expected by chance.

Not surprisingly, most hospitals are found in the center of the table with probability values between .10 and .90, indicating that it would be inappropriate to identify them as being better or worse than average based solely on these outcome data. On the other hand, more hospitals appear in the extreme categories than would be expected purely by chance, suggesting that some hospitals, in fact, have significantly better or worse outcomes. Among the twenty-nine very low-volume hospitals in table 8.2, five had death rates greater than what would be expected purely by chance 97.5 percent of the time.

In contrast, none of the very low-volume hospitals exhibited better than expected performance at usual levels of statistical significance. However, before one assumes that low-volume catheterization units cannot have better than average outcomes, one must recognize that the

TABLE 8.2. Distribution of Hospitals by Results for Cardiac Catheterization Patients

Volume per Year	Probability that Observed = Expected Outcome	Very Low 1–200	Low 201–400	Medium 401–500	High 501–750	Very High 750+	Total
Outcomes much better than expected	< 0.025	0	1	0	0	5	6
	0.025–0.050	0	0	1	1	2	4
	0.051–0.100	0	0	1	0	3	4
	0.101–0.500	6	21	7	12	6	52
	0.501–0.900	15	19	5	11	6	56
	0.901–0.950	3	1	0	0	0	4
	0.951–0.975	0	1	1	1	0	3
Outcomes much worse than expected	> 0.975	5	6	4	2	3	20
Total		29*	49	19	27	25	149

*Two hospitals, with one and two patients each, are excluded.

Note: For each hospital, the probability is calculated using the binomial distribution. To smooth the results associated with the occurrence of integral values, the calculated probability is the average of results from the binomial for the probabilites that the observed number of deaths, and one plus the observed number of deaths, would occur given the number of patients and the mortality rate expected based upon the age and diagnoses of the patients.

nature of the binomial distribution makes it an impossibility for such hospitals to record performances significantly better than expected. With a death rate of 1 percent, and with the maximum number of patients for this category (200) there would be only 2.0 deaths per year if the hospital's performance was just average, and we would expect to observe zero deaths about 14 percent of the time owing to random variation. Since fewer than zero deaths cannot be observed, it is impossible to reliably identify low-volume hospitals as having better than average performance for patients with low mortality rates unless several years of data are pooled.

In the intermediate-volume categories for cardiac catheterization, an occasional hospital is identified as having better than expected outcomes, but it is important to recall that some such observations can occur by chance. This finding is consistent with the grouped results indicating that hospitals with intermediate volumes collectively have average performance. On the other hand, five of the twenty-five very high-volume hospitals have much better than expected performance. (The probability value of .025 means that less than one hospital [25 × .025 = .625] should present such good results merely by chance.) Yet the fact that three very high-volume hospitals had substantially worse than expected performance suggests that high volume does not guarantee success.

The use of hospital-specific probabilities means that we can narrow our focus from all 151 hospitals to the 23 with results outside the .025 to .975 range or the 33 outside the .05 to .95 range. This does not mean that all hospitals with outcomes within the confidence interval are truly average performers, but if one had to choose just a few hospitals for detailed review, it is the outliers that might best be put at the top of the list. In particular, one would expect about 15 hospitals to fall outside the .05 to .95 range just by chance, even if all were truly average performers. Thus about half the outliers identified on the basis of one year's outcomes are there by chance, so one should view the finding of significantly "better" or "worse" than expected performance not as a final classification, but as a yellow flag that warrants investigation. For example, table 8.3 presents some of the characteristics of those hospitals with significantly higher and lower than expected death rates. The table also includes results for some hospitals that might stand out to the casual observer. While in a real situation, one would have substantially more data available about each hospital, even this limited information is instructive.

Hospital A has a death rate more than six times what would be expected based on its case mix, which is highly unlikely as a chance occurrence, even with only 70 patients. The hospital has only one

TABLE 8.3. Characteristics of Selected Hospitals

	Number of Patients	Cardiac Catheterization Deaths	Observed/ Expected Deaths	Expected Death Rate	Probability	Beds	Neighboring Hospitals	Cath. Labs	Medical-school Affiliated
A	70	6	6.261	0.0137	0.99997	100	0	0	No
B	161	24	6.179	0.0241	0.99999	200	26	12	No
C	423	1	0.163	0.0145	0.03492	500	7	6	No
D	474	0	0.000	0.0051	0.19653	300	8	2	No
E	1,036	27	1.631	0.0159	0.99539	600	29	7	Yes

hundred beds and is not affiliated with a medical school. It has no neighboring hospitals within fifteen miles, and it is possible there may be few alternatives available within any reasonable distance. In contrast, hospital B is within fifteen miles of twenty-six other hospitals, twelve of which have catheterization labs, so it is difficult to justify its poor performance on the grounds of access. With 24 deaths among 161 patients, hospital B is likely to be quickly chosen for review, but what about hospital E with 27 deaths among 1,036 patients? This is a large, medical school–affiliated hospital, with many neighboring facilities, yet its death rate is almost two-thirds above what would be expected from its case mix, and such outcomes are extremely unlikely by chance given the large number of patients. It may be the case, however, that careful review of the patients' charts, such as in a mortality and morbidity conference, will uncover risk factors that account for the deaths and are not included in the risk measure.

Probabilities are also useful in evaluating what may appear to be very favorable death rates. The performance of hospital D, with zero deaths among almost 500 patients, at first glance appears superior to that of hospital C with one death among about 400 patients. However, hospital D's case mix is at substantially lower risk of death and its zero death rate is not significantly different than what would be expected by chance.

CONCLUSION AND POLICY IMPLICATIONS

These data demonstrate that for a procedure such as cardiac catheterization, one can observe, using readily available case-abstract data for a large sample of hospitals, an inverse relation between the number of patients treated in a hospital and their subsequent mortality. Identifying the causal factors is a complex task that is the subject of other research. Recognition of such a relationship may suggest to some that patients should be directed away from low-volume institutions and toward high-volume hospitals. However, even if this were an appropriate conclusion for policy purposes, there is much more to consider than just volume. Some low-volume hospitals have quite good outcomes and some high-volume hospitals have outcomes significantly worse than expected for their case mix. In designing policies in response to these findings, it is important to distinguish policies that are appropriately directed toward groups or classes of institutions and those directed toward individual hospitals.

The observation of a general relation between volume and outcome suggests that if there is no way to obtain better, more specific data, then volume may be a useful indicator for certain situations. For example, if general advice is to be given to the public about cardiac catheterization, it would not be inappropriate to mention that institutions with higher volumes generally have better outcomes than those with very low volumes, that is, fewer than 200 procedures per year. Third-party payers seeking selective contracts may choose to negotiate only with high-volume centers, both because their outcomes in general are better and because even if low-volume centers have good results, it cannot be proven because of the wide confidence intervals. At low volumes, even an observed zero death rate is consistent with a substantially elevated true mortality rate. On the other hand, high-volume centers occasionally have significantly poor results, and such institutions should be avoided in selective contracting. Similarly, hospital malpractice carriers might want to take volume into account in adjusting their premiums if they find that claims experience is related to volume. In each instance, the recommendations are based upon general guidelines that are appropriate for probabilistic situations.

If one needs to refer a specific patient for a procedure, much more information than volume is usually available, and should be used. For example, a certain physician or medical center may have a particularly good reputation in the area and be recognized as being the place to go for extremely complicated cases. This implies that any strategy designed to influence existing referral patterns must proceed with caution in the identification of the preferred hospitals.

The situation is even more complex if one is undertaking a review of hospital performance to assess quality of care such as is mandated for peer-review organizations. The inherent variability in patient outcomes means that death rates even several times the expected value may not be significantly different from the norm. More important, the observation of zero deaths may provide little useful information if the expected death rate is low or the number of patients small.

The data presented in this chapter refer to in-hospital death rates following cardiac catheterization, but the general observations apply to any outcomes with similar rates of occurrence. In general, if the rate of adverse outcomes is substantially higher than 1 percent, such as the 16 percent death rate for acute myocardial infarction, then it is easier to identify good or poor performance with some degree of statistical confidence. On the other hand, diagnoses and procedures with very high death rates often involve extremely ill patients for whom the underlying clinical factors dominate physician or hospital performance, and few hospitals have enough patients to identify significantly better or worse results. However, one need not be limited to the analysis of mortality. Rates of postoperative complications, infections, or readmissions are similar to the range explored here of about 1 to 15 percent.

It is inherently more difficult to identify worse than expected performance in hospitals with low volumes because the confidence intervals are so wide. This does not mean, however, that it is fruitless to monitor low-volume hospitals. For example, by pooling several years of data, one can accumulate enough patient observations to reduce confidence intervals to a useful range. Similarly, one may be able to pool patients undergoing related procedures while including controls for the risks of each procedure to increase the sample size.

Once the limitations of small numbers of patients and infrequent occurrences are recognized, there are still roles for routinely collected data in evaluating hospital outcomes. Third-party payers might selectively choose to contract only with hospitals providing outcome measures and reject those with significantly poor results. Routinely collected data can be used as an indicator of where more detailed case review is likely to uncover real problems. If abstracts are to be used as indicators, then it is appropriate to cast a wider, rather than a narrower, net, or in statistical terms, it is preferable to have many false positives at the first stage in order to minimize the number of false negatives. Thus tables 8.4 and 8.5 identify for various combinations of volumes and probabilities the 80 percent confidence intervals instead of the more conventional 90 or 95 percent intervals. These are designed to be somewhat conservative, and they identify the points that are above what would be expected by chance 10 percent of the time and below what would be expected by chance 10 percent of the time.

In table 8.4 are the minimum number of deaths that would have to be observed to reject the null hypothesis that outcomes in a given hospital are not different than the overall average rate. For example, if there is an expected death rate of 15 percent, such as for abdominal aortic aneurysm, at least 6 deaths would have to be observed among 20 patients to indicate significantly poor results at the .10 level. If only 5 deaths are observed, even though the calculated death rate of 25 percent is substantially above the expected rate of 15 percent, it is not statistically significant.

In table 8.5 are the maximum number of deaths consistent with significantly good outcomes, again at the 10 percent level. For example, the observation of no deaths among 20 patients with a 15 percent expected death rate is likely to occur less than 10 percent of the time. The large number of cells labeled "N.P.", or not possible, are indicative of how difficult it is to identify a hospital or physician as performing significantly better than average even if no deaths are observed. For example, even a zero death rate is not significant for a hospital with 200 patients whose expected death rate is .01.

TABLE 8.4. Number of Deaths Consistent with a Statistically Significant Poor Outcome (at the 0.10 significance level)

Expected Death Rate	Number of Patients						
	5	10	20	50	100	200	500
0.001	1*	1*	1*	1*	1*	1	1
0.005	1*	1*	1*	2	2	3	6
0.01	1*	1*	2	2	3	5	9
0.05	2	2	3	6	9	15	32
0.10	2	3	5	9	15	27	60
0.15	3	4	6	12	21	38	86
0.20	3	5	7	15	26	48	113

*Zero deaths are expected to be observed more than 90 percent of the time with these combinations of death rates and patients. The observation of one death is highly unlikely by chance.

Even if a hospital is identified as having significantly better or worse than expected performance, one is not justified in either ordering champagne or demanding closure, because such results do occur by chance. Statistically significant results are not definitive but should be interpreted as warning flags that require further investigation. Those hospitals with significantly worse than expected performance may then be selected for intensive chart auditing or other appropriate quality-review activities. Similarly, before policies are designed to channel patients toward specific hospitals with apparently better than expected outcomes, or before they are even publicly identified as good performers, it is important that other types of evaluations support the designation.

If precautions are not taken before acting on outcome statistics, average performers will occasionally be mistakenly identified as being either worse or better than they truly are. (With a 90 percent confidence interval, one would expect 5 percent of truly average performers to appear to be worse than average and 5 percent to be better than average.) In the first instance, they will be incorrectly labeled as having worse than expected outcomes and libel suits might ensue. In the second instance, patients may be inappropriately redirected toward hospitals with performance not truly better than average, and there may be some liability for worse outcomes than would have occurred had the shift not taken place.

In spite of these statistical caveats, it is quite reasonable to use large data sets to examine general patterns of performance such as the relation between volume and outcome. Such results might be useful to malpractice carriers in rate setting or to third-party payers seeking to limit their negotiations to high-quality institutions. Furthermore, much

TABLE 8.5. Maximum Number of Deaths Consistent with Statistically Significant Good Outcomes (at the 0.10 significance level)

Expected Death Rate	Number of Patients						
	5	10	20	50	100	200	500
0.001	N.P.	N.P.	N.P.	N.P.	N.P.	N.P.	N.P.
0.005	N.P.	N.P.	N.P.	N.P.	N.P.	N.P.	0
0.01	N.P.	N.P.	N.P.	N.P.	N.P.	N.P.	1
0.05	N.P.	N.P.	N.P.	0	1	5	18
0.10	N.P.	N.P.	N.P.	1	5	14	40
0.15	N.P.	N.P.	0	3	10	23	64
0.20	N.P.	N.P.	1	5	14	32	88

N.P.: Not possible to show statistically significant good outcomes for this combination of expected death rate and volume level.

of the problem identified in this chapter arises from the low death rate associated with most hospitalizations. If complications are considered, then it is possible to examine interhospital differences with smaller samples.

As the focus of attention shifts to the evaluation of individual hospital or even physician performance, much more attention needs to be paid to the unmeasured aspects of the cases and less reliance should be placed on general patterns. Hebel and others demonstrated how case-abstract data can be used as the starting point in examining why a hospital appears to have a higher death rate than its neighbors (13). They begin with overall mortality, adjust for case mix and other factors, then narrow their focus to specific diagnostic categories. However, the shift from the general to the specific means that the number of patients quickly becomes very small. The inherent variability in patient outcomes, especially if one focuses on rare events such as death, means that statistical confidence becomes increasingly difficult to attain. It would help if attention were to shift to complication rates, both in the hospital through charts and more detailed abstract review and post hospitalization through the analysis of insurance claims. Similarly, one can gain substantial confidence if the results for specific hospitals are similar year after year. Thus, while readily available data are a powerful and inexpensive guide, they can only be used to begin the process of evaluating performance of hospitals and physicians.

REFERENCES

1. Flood, A.B., Scott, W.R., and Ewy, W. Does practice make perfect? Part 1: The relation between hospital volume and outcomes for selected diagnostic categories. Med Care 22:98–114 (1984).

2. Flood, A.B., Scott, W.R., and Ewy, W. Does practice make perfect? Part 2: The relation between volume and outcomes and other hospital characteristics. *Med Care* 22:115–25 (1984).
3. Shortell, S. and LoGerfo, J. Hospital medical staff organization and quality of care: Results for myocardial infarction and appendectomy. *Med Care* 19:1041 (1981).
4. Luft, H.S., Bunker, J., and Enthoven, A. Should operations be regionalized? The empirical relation between surgical volume and mortality. *N Eng J Med* 301:1364–69 (1979).
5. Luft, H.S. The relation between surgical volume and mortality: An exploration of causal factors and alternative models. *Med Care* 18:940–59 (1980).
6. Riley, G., and Lubitz, J. Outcomes of surgery in the Medicare-aged population: Mortality after surgery. *Health Care Fin Rev* 6:103–15 (1985).
7. Farber, B., Kaiser, D. and Wenzel, R. Relation between surgical volume and incidence of postoperative wound infection. *N Eng J Med* 305:200–03 (1981).
8. Iglehart, J.K. Cutting costs of health care for the poor in California: A two-year follow-up. *N Eng J Med* 311:745–48 (1981).
9. Brinkley, J. U.S. releasing lists of hospitals with abnormal mortality rates. *New York Times,* March 12, 1986.
10. Chorlton, P. Hospital deaths vary widely in Maryland. *Washington Post,* August 13, 1982.
11. Bargmann, E., and Grove, C. Surgery in Maryland hospitals, 1979 and 1980, charges and deaths. Washington, D.C.: Public Citizen Health Research Group (1982).
12. Jacobs, P. Report cites high death rate of medicare patients, notes other problems in care. *Los Angeles Times,* March 12, 1982.
13. Hebel, J.R., Kessler, I., Mabuchi, K., and McCarter, R. Assessment of hospital performance by use of death rates. *JAMA* 248:3131–35 (1982).
14. Dranove, D. A comment on "Does practice make perfect?" *Med Care* 22:967 (1984).
15. Flood, A.B., Scott, W.R., and Ewy, W. Letter in reply to Dranove, "A comment on 'Does practice make perfect?'" *Med Care* 22:967 (1984).
16. Luft, H.S., Hunt, S.S., and Maerki, S.C. The volume-outcome relationship: Practice makes perfect or selective referral patterns? *Hlth Serv Res* 22:157–82 (1987).
17. Adams, D.F., Fraser, D.B., and Abrams, H.L. The complications of coronary arteriography. *Circulation* 48:609–18 (1973).

9 The Federal Assessment of Surgical Procedures

Jane E. Sisk, Ph.D., and Gloria Ruby, M.A.

Substantial changes in surgery have occurred since the early 1970s. Surgical techniques have been refined, new devices and materials have been developed, and certain new procedures have been performed while other procedures have been shown to be ineffective or even dangerous. Many of these developments have been facilitated by the growth of private and public third-party payment of medical care, which expanded and made more secure the market for medical products and services. This change was especially pronounced in the coverage of services in inpatient hospital settings, where most surgery took place.

This period also witnessed a growing concern about rapidly rising expenditures for medical care, and surgical procedures were often cited to exemplify excessive and otherwise inappropriate use. In response, public and private payers, including employers, have undertaken various measures intended to contain costs: review of Medicare inpatient cases by professional standards review organizations (PSROs) and more recently by utilization and quality-control peer-review organizations (PROs); changes in coverage to encourage the substitution of ambulatory for inpatient surgery; and prospective payment of hospital cases or days.

Another response by public and private payers has been closer examination of the appropriateness of technologies used to manage medical conditions. This chapter reports on those technology assessment activities, with particular emphasis on those pertaining to surgery. The first section presents an overview of the diffusion of surgical procedures during the 1970s and early 1980s. The next section reviews selected federal activities to assess medical technologies, including surgery. In conclusion, we consider the current status of technology assessment and changes as a result of heightened concern about cost containment.

RECENT DIFFUSION OF SURGICAL PROCEDURES

Although there was little change during the 1970s and early 1980s in hospital discharges for surgery overall, this stability masked the substantial changes that occurred for certain age groups and for certain procedures. Surgical discharge rates for elderly people rose far more than for other age groups, whose rates changed little or even fell. At the same time, average lengths of stay for elderly people were falling, from about fourteen days in 1973 to about eleven days in 1983. Lengths of stay rose only for children under fifteen years.

These changes have been ascribed to advances in surgical techniques and in associated medical practices and devices, especially those for chronic conditions associated with aging (1). After analyzing trends in eleven surgical procedures from 1971 to 1981, Sloan and Valvona concluded that technological change accounted for almost all of the observed decrease in lengths of stay in more than 500 hospitals (2).*

A more detailed analysis of ten diagnoses treated at a San Francisco tertiary care hospital found that resource use remained similar between 1972 and 1982 for patients with most diagnoses (3). Lengths of stay fell significantly for acute myocardial infarction, cataract extraction, and acute asthma and rose significantly for infants with respiratory distress syndrome and for kidney transplants. But substitution of surgery for medical treatment and application of new diagnostic and therapeutic technologies in some cases offset these decreases. For example, coronary artery bypass surgery, which was performed on no myocardial infarct patients in 1972, was performed on 9 percent of them in 1982. Similarly, only 2 percent of acute myocardial infarct patients received coronary artery catheterization in 1977, but 36 percent did in 1982.

Scitovsky's update of costs of treatment for sixteen conditions in a California hospital also found small differences between 1971 and 1981 costs for many conditions (4). The major cost-saving change was a further decline in hospital lengths of stay. But the use of new expensive technologies, such as coronary bypass surgery for myocardial infarction, and greater use of existing expensive technologies, such as delivery by cesarean section, increased during the period.

The effects of changing techniques, and specifically surgery, on health outcomes were more equivocal. Showstack and colleagues found no improvement in in-hospital survival in any of the patient groups studied. Scitovsky pointed out that reduced lengths of stay reduces

---

*Any error in predicting the actual decline in stay was combined with the time trend in the category of technological change.

exposure to nosocomial infections, but the new techniques for treating breast cancer and myocardial infarcts and greater use of cesarean sections have not been clearly associated with improvements in mortality or morbidity.

Great variations have been found in the use of both surgical and medical procedures. For example, coronary artery bypass surgery for elderly Medicare beneficiaries in thirteen areas varied from 7 to 23 per 10,000 beneficiaries (5). Researchers have been unable to explain the wide variations or to clarify whether high rates are associated with excessive use or low rates with insufficient use or whether the different rates are appropriate for these areas. At the same time, it is noteworthy that enrollees of prepaid group practices, a type of health maintenance organization (HMO), have had lower surgical rates than comparison populations for decades, apparently without suffering great adverse effects on health (6–7).

During the past decade, substantial changes have been occurring in the organizational settings in which surgery is delivered. About 20 percent of surgery was performed on an ambulatory basis in 1982. Surgical procedures in hospital outpatient departments have since increased as inpatient procedures have declined, and, according to a survey published in 1985, 74 percent of hospitals were planning to add to or expand outpatient surgery programs (8).Freestanding ambulatory surgical centers are also growing. From the first one in 1970, the number had grown to over 300 by 1984 (9). An estimated half a million operations are performed in these facilities (10). These centers, however, account for only about 2 percent of total surgery, including ambulatory and inpatient procedures (8).

These organizational changes most likely reflect developments in both technology and financing. For example, changes in surgical techniques and medical devices have enabled cataract surgery to be performed much more quickly and safely (11). The development of extremely sharp needles, very fine sutures, and intraoperative keratometers for measuring corneal curvature has facilitated more effective wound closure. Surgical microscopes have enabled surgeons performing extracapsular cataract extraction to increase the precision of their measurements through enhanced vision and improved depth perception. In addition, the introduction of viscoelastic substances during cataract surgery in the early 1980s has allowed ophthalmologists to protect delicate intraocular structures and to maintain the normal shape of the eye, while still permitting the good visual capabilities needed for intraocular manipulations (11). A consequence of new technological developments has been that cataract surgery may be safely performed on an ambulatory basis. Changes in lasers, anesthesiology, and endoscopy have also contributed to the performance of more surgery on an ambulatory basis (8).

In addition to technological developments, changes in payment policies have encouraged the movement of surgery from inpatient to ambulatory settings in both the private and public sectors. However, the nature of the encouragement of ambulatory surgery in the private sector is not clear. There has been no systematic data collection on the extent to which private third-party payers simply reimburse for or actively encourage ambulatory surgery. Some insurance carriers maintain lists of procedures that will only be reimbursed if performed on an ambulatory basis; others simply provide information about the availabilty of the coverage without taking an active role in encouraging it. Some carriers have tried to increase the incentives for physicians to perform surgery in an ambulatory setting by increasing the level of outpatient reimbursement relative to that of inpatient surgery (12).

In the public sector, legislation in 1981 permitted Medicare to pay for certain procedures in freestanding ambulatory surgical centers. The Omnibus Reconciliation Act provides incentive to physicians to encourage their provision of ambulatory surgery. If physicians elect to use a surgical center and take assignment, they are paid 100 percent of their reasonable charge without regard to deductibles. Usual Medicare payment for ambulatory services is 80 percent after the deductible is met.

More important, in late 1983 Medicare began paying for hospital operating expenses on the basis of diagnosis-related groups, which entail a fixed payment for each diagnosis regardless of the length of stay and the cost or number of specific services used. This prospective payment method gives providers a financial incentive to shift surgery and other care to ambulatory settings such as hospital outpatient departments, where physicians and facilities have continued to be paid more for additional and more expensive services.

SELECTED FEDERAL ASSESSMENT ACTIVITIES

"Medical technology" refers to drugs, devices, and procedures and to organizational and support systems within which they are delivered. Technology assessment in the medical field has come to signify any evaluation of a technology, especially regarding its efficacy and safety. Comprehensive technology assessments examine the intended, unintended, and uncertain implications of a technology, including benefits, risks, costs, and other economic and social effects. Although activities and organizations to evaluate medical technologies have grown over the past decade, surgical procedures clearly remain the least regulated and least likely to be assessed of all the medical technologies used in clinical care. To some extent, this situation stems from the fact that surgical procedures are dependent on individual surgeons, who often change slightly an existing procedure or introduce a new one. Furthermore, the methodologies in place for assessments of surgical procedures are expensive and time consuming. Most often they do not compare procedures for a particular condition, and they pose serious conceptual, practical, ethical, and economic difficulties (13).

Only if the surgery involves a new device or drug is it subject to premarketing approval by the Food and Drug Administration (FDA), and only if the procedure is substantially different from existing ones is it likely to be scrutinized for coverage by third-party payers. Nonetheless, a wide assortment of assessment activities examine surgical procedures. Some institutions, for example, the National Institutes of Health, assess surgical procedures without a formal means to enforce their recommendations. Instead, they rely on information dissemination as a persuasive mechanism. Others, such as the Veterans Administration, assess surgical procedures for a limited audience. Recently, primarily in response to the publicity and costs associated with transplantation, a number of states, including New York, have undertaken an evaluation role. In addition to the federal and state governments, assessments are carried out in the private sector both by nonprofit and profit-making organizations. For example, the National Blue Cross/Blue Shield Association and a number of its state plans, including Massachusetts and California, have active assessment programs. A large number of medical associations (such as the American College of Physicians), members of the drug industry, policy research groups, and provider groups are also involved in evaluations.

National Institutes of Health, Department of Health and Human Services

The National Institutes of Health (NIH) evaluates technologies in the course of supporting clinical trials. The National Heart, Lung, and Blood Institute and the National Cancer Institute have been the largest supporters of such trials at the NIH. Studies have been funded through the National Heart, Lung, and Blood Institute to evaluate coronary artery surgery and through the National Cancer Institute to evaluate treatments for breast cancer, including alternative surgical procedures (13). Except for the drug industry, the NIH is the single largest supporter of clinical trials in the United States. The NIH obligated $235.4 million in fiscal year 1984 and $275.7 million in fiscal year 1985 for clinical trials (14). The percentage of the NIH budget allocated to assessments of surgical procedures is not available, largely because of variations among NIH bureaus, institutes, and divisions in budget categories and defining terms. Resources devoted to evaluating surgeries vary among the institutes. Most of the randomized controlled trials in cancer research are of chemotherapeutic agents. Surgery has been tested far less often. The National Heart, Lung, and Blood Institute has sponsored preventive trials and therapeutic trials related to cardiovascular disease and has focused on surgery as well as beta-blocking and antithrombotic drugs as therapeutic agents (13).

The NIH is also engaged in technology evaluation through the consensus development conferences that are sponsored by its Office of Medical Applications of Research. These conferences are intended to ease the transfer of technology and study results from research to clinical practice. The separate institutes of the NIH suggest topics for which they believe sufficient information exists to resolve certain questions. The consensus development panel, whose members are chosen to represent relevant medical disciplines and analytical expertise, reviews the literature and conference presentations and issues a statement, which is distributed by the NIH and selected medical journals.

The sparseness of rigorous information on surgical procedures is reflected in the topics chosen for the consensus development meetings. Since 1977, surgeries have been the focus of only a small proportion of the conferences. Surgical procedures considered were dental implants, indications for tonsillectomy and adenoidectomy, surgical treatment of morbid obesity, the management of primary breast cancer as a local disease, intraocular lens implantation, removal of third molars, childbirth by cesarean delivery, coronary bypass surgery, and hip joint replacement. The last major surgery discussed was liver transplantation in June 1983. Of the seven meetings held in the latter part of 1986 and in 1987, none was completely devoted to a surgical procedure and only one—the treatment of nonmetastic prostate cancer—considered surgery as a treatment modality (15).

The ability of the consensus conferences to affect practice patterns has been questioned. For example, a consensus development conference in 1980 expressed concern over the trend of rising cesarean birth rates and developed recommendations that were expected to lead to their decrease. Although the report of the conference was published as a monograph and summaries and specific recommendations appeared in the two leading obstetric and gynecological journals, cesarean section deliveries continued to rise for the five years after the conference (16).

Food and Drug Administration, Department of Health and Human Services

The Food and Drug Administration (FDA) administers laws that require manufacturers or suppliers of drugs and, since 1976, medical devices to receive approval for new products before they are marketed commercially. Although surgical (and medical) procedures are not explicitly regulated by this process, they are affected to the extent that they rely on devices or drugs.

Devices found by the FDA to be substantially equivalent to ones marketed before the 1976 law may be marketed by the manufacturer. Implantable pacemakers are an example. Otherwise, the device must go through a premarketing approval process. Until the FDA conveys premarketing approval, a device manufacturer may not sell the new device for a profit.

If a manufacturer wishes to undertake clinical studies to develop the requisite information on efficacy and safety, it must receive approval for proposed investigations from an institutional review board and, depending on the risk posed by use of the device, an "investigational device exemption" from the FDA itself. Intraocular lenses, which are inserted after 80 percent of cataract extractions (11), were the subject of such a study in the late 1970s. In fact, from 1977 to 1982, ophthalmology had the highest number of premarket approvals (47 percent of the total) and investigational device exemptions for devices that posed a significant risk (28 percent of the total) (17). Cardiovascular devices, which include heart valves and artificial hearts as well as pacemakers, also had sizeable numbers of investigational device exemptions and premarket approvals.

The FDA's evaluation of devices is limited to deciding whether the efficacy and safety of the device conform to the claims of the manufacturer in its suggested labeling. Thus the FDA does not decide on the appropriate use of the device, including its substitution for or combination with other technologies. The agency does require manufacturers to report hazards that are detected after marketing begins and may recall devices considered unsafe.

Office of Health Technology Assessment, Department of Health and Human Services

Assessment for coverage and payment purposes is the only formal review for safety and efficacy received by surgical procedures. In the public sector, the Office of Health Technology Assessment (OHTA) of the National Center for Health Services Research and Health Care Technology Assessment (NCHSR) evaluates surgical procedures and other medical technologies in response to requests from the Health Care Financing Administration (HCFA), which administers the Medicare program. In addition to its evaluation, the OHTA also provides recommendations to the HCFA about the appropriateness of providing coverage for the assessed technology, and the HCFA makes the coverage decision.

Evaluating the health benefits and risks of specific technologies has become an established part of arriving at decisions about new or unestablished medical technologies that are being considered for coverage for payment under Medicare. These assessments assume widespread importance in that many third-party payers in the private sector rely on the HCFA's coverage decisions concerning surgical and other technologies for their coverage and reimbursement decisions. Ironically, the lack of an assessment by the OHTA of a diffused technology is also of importance to private-sector third-party payers. Although heart transplantation has been recognized as an acceptable surgical procedure in the medical community for quite some time, the costs of the procedure have delayed a Medicare decision concerning payment. Other payers have been forced to make their own coverage decision about heart transplantation because the OHTA's assessment has not been publically released.

The OHTA's full assessment of a specific technology requires six to eighteen months for completion. Anywhere from seventeen evaluations (in 1985) to twenty-six evaluations (in 1982 and 1984) are completed annually (18). Twenty-one of the ninety-eight evaluations completed from 1981 to 1984 were of surgical procedures (19). In addition, numerous evaluations of technologies included surgical techniques but did not focus on the procedure, for example, the use of electrocardiography monitoring during open heart surgery.

The information for an assessment is garnered from a wide spectrum of sources. In order to hear from all interested parties, the OHTA advertises an impending assignment in the *Federal Register* and places notices in professional and trade publications. The OHTA also contacts federal agencies, the American Medical Association, and relevant specialty societies and interested manufacturers for information on the technology being evaluated.

The OHTA staff of eight professionals synthesizes and analyses the collected evidence. The types of acceptable information range from qualified medical opinions derived from personal experience to well-designed clinical studies. Although the OHTA's guidelines emphasize the value of controlled clinical trials, few evaluations have had the benefit of such rigorous evidence. Indeed, of the twenty-four full assessments in 1982, only two assessments had information from randomized controlled trials (13). Only a small fraction of health care technologies (10 to 20 percent) has ever undergone clinical trials for safety and effectiveness.

Despite their rigor, randomized controlled trials can fail to answer questions of interest for OHTA evaluations. Research into more applicable methods of assessing surgical and other technologies is necessary. Congress recognized this need in the Health Promotion and Disease Prevention Amendments of 1984 (P.L. 98-551), which established the National Advisory Council on Health Care Technology Assessments to provide advice to the NCHSR and HCTA. One of its functions is to act on grants and contracts of over $50,000 for research into methods of technology assessment.

Although Medicare beneficiaries are heavy users of particular surgical procedures (20), evaluations have not been performed for all covered surgeries. The OHTA assessments conducted thus far have examined only a minute percentage of the thousands of surgical and other technologies reimbursable under Medicare. In recognition of this situation, the OHTA has recently embarked on a coordinated effort with the HCFA to assess established technologies. Three covered technologies have been selected for assessment, two of which are surgical procedures. The two surgeries—extracranial-intracranial arterial bypass for ischemic stroke and carotid endarterectomy—vary in the availabilty of rigorous information on their effectiveness and safety.

Extracranial-intracranial (EC-IC) arterial bypass for ischemic stroke was introduced sixteen years ago, and its effectiveness was suggested by a series of uncontrolled studies and case-series reports (21). Although the procedure is covered for payment by Medicare, an assessment of the procedure was stimulated by a recent international, multicenter study that concluded that there were no indications for the procedure in the study group as a whole or in any of the subgroups that the investigators identified (22). The researchers concluded that EC-IC arterial bypass does not reduce the incidence of transient ischemic attacks or the risk of ischemic stroke in patients with atherosclerotic occlusive disease of the brain.

The effectiveness of carotid endarterectomy is not clear. This procedure is covered by Medicare and is widely diffused—119,000 procedures were performed in 1983 (23)—although professional opinions have varied about indications for its use (24) and there have been few conclusive data from which to draw conclusions about its advantages. The procedure has attracted public attention, and media reports have indicated that the complications of the procedure are greater than the benefits. A new retrospective review study expressed concern that the surgical mortality rate is higher than that considered as acceptable for patients with asymptomatic carotid disease and suggested that many of such surgeries could be unnecessary (25). The authors concluded that a more conservative approach to asymptomatic patients is warranted until evidence from randomized controlled trials as to the therapeutic value of carotid endarterectomy is available. Since there are inadequate data upon which to base an assessment, the OHTA is considering the use of HCFA claims data to determine the effects of the procedure (19).

Veterans Administration

Through its Cooperative Studies Program, the Veterans Administration (VA) supports multicenter clinical trials within the VA Medical Care system. A formally structured process is followed to ensure the quality of the study design and implementation. The Cooperative Studies Program supports trials that involve the participation of more than one VA hospital; other clinical trials are conducted within individual VA hospitals, and the VA is involved in trials funded by other agencies, such as the NIH, and by private sources, for example, pharmaceutical companies (13).

A Technology Assessment Task Force was formed within the VA in October of 1985 to prepare a comprehensive plan for technology assessment within the organization (26). Although the plan, completed in the fall of 1986, emphasizes equipment for initial implementation, it also discusses the need for assessments of pacemakers, transplants, and artificial organs.

Office of Technology Assessment, U.S. Congress

A staff arm of Congress, the Office of Technology Assessment (OTA), conducts studies related to science and technology policy that are requested by congressional committees. OTA thus has no ongoing responsibility to assess specific technologies, including surgical procedures. But in the course of an examination of health policy or in response to a specific request, OTA may evaluate specific technologies. Such OTA assessments typically review evidence regarding the technology's efficacy and safety and consider its appropriate role in medical care. The studies have also examined costs, ethics, personnel requirements, and other social implications, but often in less depth. Examples relating to surgery are operations for breast cancer, the artificial heart, and joint replacements. Other studies examined technologies such as extracorporeal shock-wave lithotripsy, which can substitute for surgery, and the immunosuppressive drug cyclosporine, which is used in conjunction with transplantation. Some cost-effectiveness analyses have been performed, but none regarding surgery.

Prospective Payment Assessment Commission

The formation of the Prospective Payment Commission (ProPac) mandated with the passage of the Social Security amendments of 1983 (P.L. 98-21) initiated a new government involvement in medical technology assessment. ProPac is an independent commission of experts appointed by the director of OTA. Its basic responsibility is to make recommendations to the secretary of Health and Human Services and the Congress regarding the need for adjustments to Medicare's DRG-based prospective payment system for inpatient hospital services. In order to do so, ProPac must identify and evaluate evidence on the safety, efficacy, and cost-effectiveness of new and existing medical technologies. ProPac is also required to assess more general changes in the health care system affecting Medicare beneficiaries, including regional variations in medical practice and lengths of hospital stay, giving special attention to treatment patterns for conditions that appear to involve costly or inappropriate services not adding to the quality of care.

ProPac, like most of the federal organizations discussed previously, has not stressed surgical procedures in its evaluations. In its April 1986 report to Congress, ProPac included recommendations for amending a number of diagnosis-related groups that involved a surgical procedure (27). The commission recommended reclassifying pacemaker cases based on the type of pacemaker, reclassifying pacemaker replacement cases depending upon the medical diagnosis, assigning implantable defibrillator cases to a unique DRG, assigning cases involving the implantation of a penile prosthesis to a unique DRG, and reclassifying a series of upper-extremity procedures with and without joint prosthesis into what they perceived as more appropriate DRGs. There was no evaluation of a surgical procedure per se. The commission did, however, recommend that utilization and quality control peer-review organizations (PROs) be required to review and monitor the quality of care and outcome of ambulatory surgery for selected patients and procedures (27).

Council on Health Care Technology, Institute of Medicine

A joint federal government–private sector activity is underway at the Institute of Medicine, part of the National Academy of Sciences. The proliferation of medical technologies and the absence of an organization to coordinate and complement existing technology assessment activities prompted the Institute of Medicine (IOM) to appoint a committee to develop a plan for a technology assessment organization. The plan recommended the creation of a nonpartisan consortium based in the private sector and supported by both governmental and private funds.

The Health Promotion and Disease Prevention Amendments of 1984 (P.L. 99-117) carried through the IOM's recommendations by mandating the establishment of the Council on Health Care Technology by the IOM/National Academy of Sciences.

The fifteen members of the council were appointed by the National Academy of Sciences in March 1986. The council is funded by a federal grant of $500,000 for the first year, which is to be followed by federal grants—$750,000 for the second and for the third year—if matched by twice the amount from nonfederal sources. Fundraising efforts have started and private-sector groups are responding.

One of the primary mandated functions of the council is to serve as a clearinghouse for information on health care technologies and assessment in order to assist other organizations. Rather than creating a model like those currently in operation, the council is developing a strategy for a "user-generated," "user-friendly" clearinghouse. Its other mandated activities include

—the collection and analysis of data concerning specific health care technologies,
—the identification of needs in assessment of technologies and research on assessment methods
—the development and evaluation of assessment criteria and methods
—the promotion of education, training, and technical assistance in the use of assessment methods and results
—the initiation, coordination, and funding of assessments

Specific concerns related to surgery entail the dearth of information on controversial surgical procedures and the concept of limiting the application of some technologies, such as coronary artery bypass surgery, to centers of competence. Although activities directed to these issues have not yet been initiated, the council is indirectly addressing the problem of insufficient information on surgical procedures by emphasizing the development of alternative methods of technology assessment. Although randomized clinical trials offer an excellent approach to assessments of surgical procedures, they are often expensive, time-consuming, and lag behind changes in practice. Furthermore, they often do not compare competing technologies but address only the safety and effectiveness of a new individual technology.

CONCLUSION

Evaluation of surgical procedures in the federal sector is scanty and flawed. Although information and evaluation is insufficient for medical technology as a whole, the dearth of activities related to surgery is particularly striking. Of all federal agencies, the OHTA is the most likely to examine the safety and efficacy of surgical procedures. Assessments of such procedures by other federal agencies have been limited and have often addressed devices that are associated with surgery rather than a surgical procedure per se.

The OHTA's evaluation of surgeries and other technologies has been limited to evaluations of safety and efficacy. But even limited to these two factors, evaluation is difficult. Basic to the problem of assessment is the difficulty of obtaining data on safety and efficacy for new technologies. In the case of surgical procedures, rigorous data are sparse even for established procedures, including tonsillectomy, appendectomy, and hysterectomy.

Randomized clinical trials are considered to be the most rigorous method of establishing safety and efficacy, but they have weaknesses with respect to assessment of surgical procedures. A surgical procedure is not static or contained like a drug. It often changes over time and is not independent of the method but is related to the skill of the surgeon, which may improve with practice (13). As with other technologies, the ethical questions associated with withholding possibly efficacious treatment for life-threatening conditions are serious.

Factors besides efficacy and safety that are necessary for the full evaluation of a technology—cost, ethical, and other societal factors—are not explicitly examined by the OHTA. The VA has been considering cost in the course of its cooperative trials. Although the legality of considering cost in Medicare coverage decisions is disputed, information on cost and other factors is certainly important for decisions by health care providers about surgical facilities and personnel and by third-party payers about coverage and payment rates.

Growing concern about containing medical expenditures has stimulated greater attention to technology assessment in the private as well as the public sector. Cost consciousness is spreading from insurers and employers who pay for medical services to providers who perform the services and ultimately to suppliers who develop and market medical products. Manufacturers of drugs and medical devices are increasingly producing evaluations of the relative costs of their products compared with alternatives. Large health care delivery systems, such as the Kaiser-Permanente Medical Care Program, and hospital chains are also evaluating technologies. For a health maintenance organization such as Kaiser-Permanente, the major issue is often whether to purchase services such as open-heart surgery from providers outside their organization or to acquire the necessary personnel and facilities and to perform it internally.

However, one cannot expect the slack in surgical evaluations to be taken up by private sector activities. The large organizations that are generating information are likely to consider it proprietary, because disseminating it might aid their competitors. And without external review of study design and procedure, suppliers' analyses would suspect because of a possible conflict of interest.

Evaluations of surgical procedures, like those of other technologies, are typical public goods: the information is in everyone's interest to have, but in no one's interest to pay to develop alone. The organization with the greatest current potential is the IOM's Council on Health Care Technology, but its budget is woefully inadequate for the task. Only a much more sizable infusion of funds and development of research methodology, perhaps by the NCHSR or the IOM, could begin to produce the information needed for surgical assessments.

REFERENCES

1. Lubitz, J., Riley, G., and Newton, M. Outcomes of surgery among the Medicare aged: Mortality after surgery. *Health Care Fin* 6:103–15 (1985).
2. Sloan, F.A., and Valvona, J. Why has hospital length of stay declined? An evaluation of alternative theories. *Soc. Sci and Med* 22:69–73 (1986).
3. Showstack, J.A., Stone, M.H., and Schroeder, S.A. The role of changing clinical practices in the rising costs of hospital care. *N Eng J Med* 313:1201–7 (1985).
4. Scitovsky, A.A., Changes in the costs of treatment of selected illnesses, 1971–1981. *Med Care* 23:1345–57 (1985).
5. Chassin, M.R., Brook, R.H., Park, R.E., et al. Variations in the use of medical and surgical services by the medicare population. *N Eng J Med* 314:285–89 (1986).
6. Luft, H.S. *Health Maintenance Organizations: Dimensions of Performance.* New York: John Wiley and Sons (1981).
7. Manning, W.G., Leibowitz, A., Goldberg, G.A., et al. A controlled trial of the effect of a prepaid group practice on use of services. *N Eng J Med* 310:1505–10 (1984).
8. Surgery proposed for outpatient rates. *Washington Report on Medicine and Health* 39, Sept. 2, 1985.
9. Ermann, D., and Gabel, J. The changing face of American health care: Multihospital systems, emergency centers, and surgical centers. *Med Care* (in press).
10. SMG Marketing Group. *Mod Hlthcare,* May 15, 1984, as cited in *Biomedical Business International* 7:96 (1984).
11. Garrison, L.P., and Yamashiro, S.M. *Background Paper on Cataract Surgery and Physician Payment under the Medicare Program.* Prepared for the Office of Technology Assessment, U.S. Congress (1985).

12. Fox, P.D., Goldbeck, W.B., and Speis, J.J. *Synthesis of Private Sector Health Care Initiatives.* Report for the Office of the Assistant Secretary for Planning and Evaluation, U.S. Department of Health and Human Services, Washington, D.C. (1984).
13. U.S. Congress, Office of Technology Assessment, *The Impact of Randomized Clinical Trials on Health Policy and Medical Practice.* Washington, D.C.: U.S. Government Printing Office (1983).
14. Institute of Medicine. *Assessing Medical Technologies.* Washington, D.C.: National Academy Press (1985).
15. Elliott, J., Office of Medical Applications of Research, National Institutes of Health, Bethesda, MD. Personal communication, June 24, 1986.
16. Gleicher, Norbert. Cesarean section rates in the United States: the short-term failure of the National Consensus Development Conference in 1980. *JAMA* 252:3273-76 (1984).
17. U.S. Department of Health and Human Services, Food and Drug Administration, unpublished data (1983). Cited in U.S. Congress, Office of Technology Assessment. *Federal Policies and the Medical Devices Industry.* Washington, D.C.: U.S. Government Printing Office (1984).
18. U.S. Department of Health and Human Services, National Center for Health Services Research and Health Care Technology Assessment. *Office of Health Technology Assessment Reports, 1981-1985: Titles and Ordering Information.* Rockville, Md. (1986).
19. Carter, E., Office of Health Technology Assessment, National Center for Health Services Research and Health Care Technology Assessment, Rockville, Md. Personal communication, June 13, 1986.
20. Burney, I., and Schieber, G. Medicare physicians' services: The composition of spending and assignment rates. *Health Care Fin Rev* 7:81-96 (1985).
21. Plum, F. Extracranial-intracranial arterial bypass and cerebral vascular disease. *N Eng J Med* 313:1221-23 (1985).
22. EC/IC Bypass Study Group. Failure of extracranial-intracranial arterial bypass to reduce the risk of ischemic stroke: Results of an international randomized trial. *N Eng J Med* 313:1191-2000 (1985).
23. American College of Surgeons. *Socioeconomic Fact Book for Surgery.* Chicago: American College of Surgeons (1986).
24. Barnett, H.J.M., Plum F., and Walton, J.N., Carotid endarterectomy—an expression of concern. *Stroke* 15:941-43 (1984).
25. Brott, T.G., Labutta, R.J., and Kempczinski, R.F. Changing patterns in the practice of carotid endarterectomy in a large metropolitan area. *JAMA* 255:2609-12 (1986).
26. Travers, E., Chairman, Task Force on Technology Assessment, Veterans Administration, Washington, D.C. Personal communication, June 14, 1986.
27. Prospective Payment Assessment Commission. *Report and Recommendations to the Secretary, U.S. Department of Health and Human Services* Washington, D.C.: U.S. Government Printing Office (1986).

28. Prospective Payment Assessment Commission. *Technical Appendixes to the Report and Recommendations to the Secretary, U.S. Department of Health and Human Services.* Vol. 2. Washington, D.C.: U.S. Government Printing Office (1985).
29. U.S. Department of Health and Human Services. *Health United States 1985.* DHHS (PHS) Pub. No. 86-1232. Hyattsville, Md. (1985).
30. U.S. Department of Health and Human Services. *Health United States 1980.* DHHS (PHS) Pub. No. 81-1232. Hyattsville, Md. (1980).

10 What Does the Future Hold?

Leslie L. Roos

Controversies regarding unnecessary surgery and the potential surplus of surgeons seem likely to remain, and perhaps intensify, in the future. The need for strategies to contain costs without adversely affecting the quality of care may continue to dominate much of the discussion of health policy. The projected increases in the supply of surgeons pose a range of problems for the financing and the quality of care. But that is only one issue; research on utilization has raised a number of additional questions.

The findings of variation in surgical rates across small hospital market areas (regardless of the country being studied) should stimulate research, both in the United States and elsewhere. The question of where surgery should be done may increase in importance as new ways of organizing health care delivery spread. More information on outcomes of even the most common surgical procedures is needed; the costs, risks, and benefits of operating, as opposed to not operating, must be better assessed. As new technologies arise, these issues are likely to become even more important. As Hampton stressed, "If investigation and treatment are to be limited we must know which investigations and which treatments are valuable and which are not" (1). Thus this chapter will consider both policy questions and research needs in the context of current and developing issues.

SUPPLY OF PHYSICIANS

The supply and distribution of physicians are, and will remain, major issues. As Rutkow and others pointed out, the supply of American

---

I gratefully acknowledge the help of the Manitoba Health Services Commission. This research was supported by National Health Research and Development Project No. 6607-1197-44 and by Career Scientist Award No. 6607-1314-48. Interpretations and viewpoints contained in this paper are my own and do not necessarily represent the opinion of either the Manitoba Health Services Commission or Health and Welfare Canada. I also wish to thank Kerry Meagher for the preparation of the manuscript.

physicians is still growing relatively rapidly (2)*. Given physicians' ability to generate demand for a substantial portion of their services, such growth will complicate both cost control and the quality of care. The supply and the orientation of surgeons and other physicians are likely to be important. Training, both formal and by example, will no doubt influence physicians' orientation. Thus Kralewski and colleagues (3) stressed the need for curriculum material "on the economics of health care effective patient care, and the functions of organizations in the provision of health services." These issues are becoming more salient to surgeons as the American health care system undergoes rapid change.

As Reinhardt (4) emphasized with regard to American cost-control efforts, decreases in one sector may be readily offset by increases elsewhere. In a fee-for-service system, "physicians' styles of practice provide sufficient elasticity to buffer most of the marketplace effects which normally impinge upon the increasing doctor-to-population ratio" (5). Although the growth in the supply of physicians is likely to have a substantial impact on health care expenditures, Perrin and Valvona (6) stressed that "current and previous studies provide little support for the idea that quality is greatly influenced by changing physician density." Improvements in the quality of care may depend much more on "focused efforts to improve the services that physicians provide" and on health promotion.

Projected increases in the supply of surgeons and other physicians cannot be justified by an aging population (7). The amount of time elderly individuals spend in hospitals and what happens to them is strongly affected by factors other than their "health needs." If more physicians would adopt a conservative, less hospital-oriented practice style (and no data suggest that the health of individuals treated under such a practice would be worse than that of individuals treated otherwise), then increasing numbers of elderly may require no increase at all in the most expensive health care resource—the hospital.

Quite apart from any pressure that the needs of the elderly population might place on the hospital sector, the projected growth in the number of physicians will place major stress on this sector. In fee-for-service medicine, physicians expect to have access to hospital beds for their patients; growth in the number of physicians alone will increase the perceived need for more beds and more expensive technology. Organizational factors, the availability of hospital beds, how physicians practice medicine, and the increase in the supply of physicians over the next several decades seem likely to influence health care costs more than will the aging of society.

---

*See also chapter 2 above.

The spread of health maintenance organizations (HMOs) and preferred provider organizations (PPOs) in the United States does show signs of generating some countervailing economic forces. The lower surgical rates associated with enrollment in prepaid group practices do not appear to have adversely affected health (8). The expanding physician supply is, however, a continuing impetus toward the delivery of more services. Several physician-related factors independent of patient health status can affect overall utilization (5,9):

—practice style
—referral patterns
—the number of physicians practicing
—patient-initiated "shopping" among physicians

The relative importance of each variable is no doubt influenced by the type of medical condition involved; factors may vary from area to area. Using Michigan data, Stano stressed that "if high utilization results from a larger number of providers becoming involved in the treatment process, a more careful examination of referral and choice decisions may answer some important questions" (9).

An increased understanding of organizational patterns and referral networks can make a major contribution to our knowledge of physician practice and small-area variations (5). In a fee-for-service system, physicians may "share" patterns as supply increases; physicians and groups of physicians have distinctive referral patterns that need to be studied more thoroughly (10).

REVIEW OF UTILIZATION

Over the next decades, several techniques of utilization review will help control hospital costs and maintain the quality of care. The following types of analyses seem likely to increase:

—case-mix adjustment using diagnosis-related groups to study length of stay
—small-area variation in rates, particularly of hospitalization for common surgical and medical conditions
—discretionary hospitalization for both surgical and medical conditions
—ambulatory versus inpatient surgery
—readmissions and other morbidity and mortality after the initial hospital stay

The utilization review methods discussed here depend on computerized data bases. Concerns about the reliability and validity of such data have often been expressed, but—given appropriate quality checks on each data set used—their potential is great (11). Using modern computer techniques to analyze large data sets facilitates research on many aspects of surgical practice (12). Work on small-area variation and on surgical outcomes has proceeded to the point that insurers and policymakers are actively involved in applying the results of this research. The flexibility of these data bases permits various research activities: adjusting the size of medical market areas, looking at the impact of physician migration on utilization, tracing referral patterns, and so on.

How should insurers and hospitals proceed with utilization review? Organizations will differ markedly in their experience with these techniques. In learning how to do such reviews, the likelihood of successful implementation of each step must be carefully considered. An organization just starting a serious review program might consider the following criteria:

1. The accessibility of the conceptual framework. Is the method easily understood by analysts, administrators, and practitioners?
2. The simplicity of data requirements. Hospital separation abstracts are usually the easiest health care data sets to work with.
3. The availability of appropriate software. Several systems are now in place to perform relevant analyses.

DRGs and Case-Mix Adjustment

Insurers, hospitals, and physicians are interested in adjusting for case mix to better compare resource use among different health care providers. Analyses based on the length of stay associated with different types of cases (such as those based on diagnosis-related groups) are probably the simplest to perform because they satisfy the three criteria noted above. Hospital separation abstracts need to be run first through a "grouper" program (such as that used to assign DRGs to ICDA-9-CM codes). Then standard statistical software (such as the SAS system or SPSS) can easily analyze the resulting data set. Because adoption of DRGs by the U.S. Medicare system has markedly changed hospital funding and may well have contributed to the slower rise in hospital costs in at least the 1983–84 period (13–14), continued efforts in improving case-mix classification seem both likely and appropriate. Related work is being directed toward classification of physician-based ambulatory encounters (15–16).

Although DRGs have been criticized on several counts (particularly clinical relevance and not accounting for enough within-DRG variance in length of stay and resource use), they seem to be "here to stay" in terms of providing a basis for Medicare payments and cost control. Incorporating other classification systems based on ICDA-9-CM do not readily improve upon the DRG coding (17–18). Although efforts are underway to improve the DRGs by incorporating co-morbidity (19), by splitting particular categories that combine inpatient and outpatient surgery (20), and by coding for severity of illness (21), changes are likely to be incremental in nature. There is considerable researcher and practitioner interest in improving case-mix adjustment (22). The extent to which improvements in case-mix adjustment can only come about through expensive changes in coding of hospital records is a controversial research issue. As discussed below, computerized data available through the reimbursement system may help provide such improvement.

Small-Area Analysis

As Wennberg, McPherson, and Caper showed, the potential for cost savings using small-area analysis appears great (23). Implementing utilization review to look at small-area variation is fairly straightforward. As stressed by Wennberg (24), major differences (up to fivefold) among small areas for a substantial number of different surgical and medical admissions are characteristically found. Overall utilization may vary markedly (often over 50 percent) among areas (25). Considerable research has been directed toward this variation; local physician (or surgeon) supply and hospital bed supply have been shown to be of some importance.

The methodology of small-area analysis has evolved and no doubt will improve further over time. Many of the suggestions by Moore in chapter 5 above have already been met. Specifically, variations in patient health status have been studied in several papers using North American research sites (26–28). The variation in patient health status has consistently been much less than the variation in many surgical rates (and in hospitalization for many medical conditions). In similar fashion, other population characteristics have been taken into account in a number of papers studying small-area variations in surgical rates (29).

Recent research on diffusion and variation has thrown some light on the physician behavior underlying small-area rates. Several Canadian studies have suggested some of the conditions by which variation is maintained, or lessened, as new procedures are adopted (10,30). If considerable care is received outside a given area, a rate can be divided into two components: the rate generated by surgery *in* this area plus the rate generated by surgery *outside* the area (typically in an urban center). In Manitoba, variation tended to be minimized when a procedure was performed in several regional centers (e.g., total hip and total knee placement) rather than in just a single metropolitan area (e.g., coronary artery bypass graft surgery). Reluctance to refer to a metropolitan center for diagnosis was reflected in a lower rate for both diagnosis and surgical treatment of cardiovascular conditions in one region well supplied with physicians.

The use of longitudinal data in a number of American studies of small-area variation (31–32) refutes Moore's criticism that such research neglects changes over time. A study of the supply of physicians, their workloads, and utilization of surgical services in rural Manitoba showed adult surgical rates to increase markedly when a surgically active physician moved into one of the areas. Among several models of physician behavior tested, the one emphasizing the importance of physician discretion provided the best fit with the data (33).

Future studies may well include more information on individual hospitals and practitioners than in the past. Recent work using data from Maine and Manitoba has focused on both hospital and physician variables and has highlighted certain hospitals (without revealing their actual names) as having worse outcomes than others (34–35). Hospitals and practitioners can also be classified in terms of the risk factors associated with the patients on whom specific operations are performed.

The cohort studies suggested by Moore will be useful if the cohorts can be defined appropriately. Previous use of the health care system (whether involving ambulatory visits or hospitalization) may not be sufficient to identify those individuals likely to have surgery. For example, one study of cholecystectomy found that 27 percent of those having surgery had fewer than two physician contacts for abdominal symptoms of gallbladder disease in the two years prior to surgery (36). These patients appear to be individuals whose physician considered the detection of stones itself to be an indication for surgery, as well as those whose stones were relatively silent until acute disease developed. For certain conditions, studies comparing groups that were treated surgically and those treated by other means may be practical. Such research has been carried out for tonsillectomy and for valve surgery (37–39).

Other approaches are also being developed. As discussed by Roos and Roos in chapter 6, significant potential exists for monitoring hospitals by using newly developed measures of discretionary hospitalization and of the underuse of ambulatory surgery. Such measures will doubtless be tested in the coming years (40).

Outcomes

Hospital-focused research is limited by the lack of ability to locate care delivered elsewhere, by problems of generalizability of findings from teaching centers, and so forth. Probably the most cost-effective tactics involve the use of large routinely collected data bases for monitoring short- and long-term outcomes. Although limited by its focus on in-hospital outcomes, chapter 8 provides an example of such research. Population-based outcome research, which permits tracing all care received (no matter where) over substantial periods of time, seems certain to increase. Such work will prove important for technology assessment, for assessing interhospital differences, and for monitoring the quality of care.

Outcome studies are highly relevant to other issues relatively unexplored in the literature. Although decision analysis has been forwarded as important for clinicians (41–42), advocates of this technique have not generally incorporated into their calculations the findings that adverse outcomes may vary by a factor of two or more, depending upon the hospital. Since the choice of appropriate therapy (surgical or medical) may often be a "close call," just taking mean estimates from the (often meager) literature on outcomes may well lead to a prosurgical bias. Thus Eisenman's summary (43) of the risks of surgery appears to underestimate the overall risks associated with such procedures as prostatectomy, coronary artery bypass graft surgery, carotid indarterectomy, and extracranial-intracranial bypass surgery (35,44–47). Such underestimates are compounded when surgery takes place at a hospital having a relatively poor performance record. A literature based on a few studies from teaching hospitals emphasizes results from generally high-quality institutions. Actual results from the wider population of hospitals are probably not as favorable.

Readmissions

Increased monitoring of readmissions also seems likely, particularly given possible incentives to discharge too early under the Medicare prospective payment system (13,48). Several research groups (Epstein and colleagues at Harvard, Goldberg and colleagues at Boston University) are actively using the computer to help identify complications after diagnostic or therapeutic procedures. Previous studies have dealt with complications resulting from three common surgical procedures (hysterectomy, cholecystectomy, and prostatectomy) (49). Complications leading to hospital readmissions are particularly important outcome measures because of the relative ease with which readmissions and accompanying diagnoses can be identified from health insurance data bases. Developing techniques for analyzing readmissions has important practical applications in facilitating the work of quality assurance committees. If the computer can identify cases with a high probability of having complications, the physician workload on such committees can be both greatly reduced and made more meaningful.

For some procedures, identifying which outcomes are complications of surgery will be difficult. This is especially true for cardiovascular surgery; to what extent is a myocardial infarction five weeks after bypass surgery a result of the operation? Readmissions and other postsurgical outcomes might be analyzed in terms of three categories: complications, other morbidity (adverse outcomes), and mortality. Some disagreement as to whether an outcome is or is not a complication can be expected. Such assessment techniques using available information systems may represent a significant advance both in helping to assess the risks of medical technologies and in judging in which hospital a given procedure should be performed.

CROSS-CUTTING ISSUES

In utilization review, several issues cut across wide-ranging concerns. One question is where surgery should be performed. Two other issues relate to improving our abilities to control for case mix efficiently and to feed information back to hospitals and providers.

Centralization

Several studies have shown both that the outcomes of many procedures are better when hospitals and physicians have experience with the particular operation and that some hospitals have significantly worse outcomes than others (34–35,50). Despite such results, an expanding supply of physicians is likely to make centralization more difficult.

Implementing a strategy of centralization of selective surgical procedures or medical treatments while preserving equality of access will take considerable thought and effort. Although American studies are lacking, some Canadian data suggest that an unwillingness to refer a patient for treatment centrally may be stronger in areas with a considerable number of specialists than in those served by general practitioners (7). Because the indications for referral often leave great discretion to the individual practitioner, local specialists may be reluctant to refer and take the chance of losing a patient to their metropolitan colleagues.

If volume and experience are important in assuring the best possible surgical outcomes, the diffusion of technology poses special difficulties for those responsible for assuring the quality of care. Surgeons wishing to learn how to perform a new, highly technical procedure obviously have to start somewhere. Since surgeons doing such new procedures can be expected to have the requisite formal qualifications, restricting access to high-volume centers will be controversial. Since some low-volume centers have relatively good results (35), such restrictions may be unfair. A number of possibilities present themselves: more stringent formal training of the surgeon, training of the entire operative team, cooperative programs involving experienced surgeons (when geographically feasible), stringent controls on the spread of technology, and so forth. The problem of maintaining the quality of health care must be addressed seriously in the years ahead.

Claims Data and Case-Mix Controls

Improving the art of case-mix control would facilitate "studies of provider productivity, prospective reimbursement, and nonexperimental studies of health outcomes" (51). As Ermann suggested in chapter 7, evaluation of ambulatory versus inpatient surgery has been hindered by the lack of appropriate case-mix controls. As noted earlier, various research groups have been trying to generate better case-mix controls (52). The demand and potential for providing risk-adjusted outcome data are great. Beyond the United States, key items of information are common across many data sets. Thus specific elements from Maine Medicare and Manitoba data have been combined and analyzed together (35). Because hospital claims (based on discharge abstracts) are both more reliable and available in more sites (provinces, states, etc.) than medical claims filed by physicians, analyses of case mix will probably focus on hospital data.

However, there are difficulties in making these changes. Overreliance on the discharge abstract generated for a given hospitalization presents a problem. Distinguishing whether "a comorbidity or complication was present on admission (i.e., preceded surgery) or occurred later in the course of the hospital stay, after surgery" may prove difficult (53). Health-status measures that rely on previous hospitalizations may provide covariates useful in exploring the associations between various health outcomes (readmission, mortality) and other independent variables (whether hospital, physician, or individual). At a time when cost and logistic constraints limit primary data collection, these computerized data ("claims") are an available and relatively inexpensive byproduct of the health care system. Population-based studies with large sample sizes are particularly facilitated by such information. Moreover, because data specific both to the individual and to the health care encounter are often available, longitudinal files can combine several types of data (e.g., hospital and physician claims) over a period of years. Finally, in addition to documenting the volume, timing, and nature of services delivered, claims contain substantial information regarding the problems for which health services are sought. Such data have supported the development of DRGs and similar classification systems.

How should such data be used for risk adjustment? Statisticians prefer construction of scales and indices; to quote Mosteller, Gilbert, and McPeek, "The potential gain from measurement offers one reason for developing scales of measurement" (54). Scales offer both increased reliability and a metric measure rather than a dichotomy; consequently the required sample size can be smaller.

On the other hand, single items make more intuitive sense to clinicians and administrators. Thus Wennberg and colleagues (35) suggested controlling for illness level by using "prior medical history variables limited to institutional events during the six-month period prior to the date of prostatectomy." Included in these events were

1. a history of having been in a nursing home or extended-care facility,
2. prior hospitalization with a diagnosis of cancer other than cancer of the prostate or bladder, and
3. prior hospitalization with a diagnosis of acute myocardial infarction, congestive heart failure, or other significant cardiopulmonary disease.

Using so many measures does heighten the difficulties of, on the one hand, attaining statistical significance by chance and, on the other, having too few cases of a certain diagnostic category to attain such significance.

Given the predictive power of covariates derived from claims data (7, 55), their further development, including comparisons with more expensive methods, should be encouraged. Such studies show how much additional data collection (record review, clinical interviews, physiologic variables) can add to case classification. No set of covariates will be perfect; covariates from claims should, however, usefully highlight institutional differences in patient comorbidity.

Feedback

Ways of feeding back the results of monitoring also need to be explored systematically. The Maine Medical Assessment Program (31) has been physician run and has fed back information to practitioners in a supportive manner. An initial goal of the program has been to bring small-area rates and lengths of stay within the range (with two or three standard deviations) of the state mean.

Wennberg (56) predicted several specific effects of monitoring of outcomes:

1. The Hawthorne effect: The general quality of care in the region will improve when physicians realize that results are being monitored.
2. A general effect: When information on outcomes for elective operations indicates that results are generally worse than reported in the literature, the rate of use of such elective operations will be reduced.
3. A specific effect: When the staffs of hospitals with worse than average outcomes learn of their situation, the quality of care will improve.

There is some evidence that monitoring and feedback of surgical rates (rather than outcomes) has had effects similar to those presented above. Both the research of Dyck and colleagues (57) on hysterectomies in Saskatchewan and the Maine Medical Assessment Project appear to have generated similar results across several procedures performed by different specialties. Specific suggestions for controlling costs and improving the quality of care should accompany feedback of the results to providers.

McAfee (58) took the position that "the success of programs that address practice variations in achieving beneficial change in physician behavior has occurred only because these data were presented to individual physicians or hospital staffs with an invitation for their analysis and input, without fear of sanction from third parties, licensure board, or a credentials committee." On the other hand, one type of intervention may be effective in some situations and not in others. Despite both a lack of supporting evidence for and consensus conferences' advice against (59) the procedure, mandatory repeat cesarean section has continued widely throughout North America (60).* When faced with such perverse patterns, insurers may wield sufficient clout to get the immediate attention of both hospital administrators and physicians. The second-opinion surgery programs provide an example of changes in delivery patterns encouraged by insurers (61).

Public release of institution-specific data on mortality and readmissions, if analyzed appropriately, need not be a bad thing. Wagner, Knaus, and Draper (62) stressed the potentially useful information provided by hospital-specific rates, particularly if better measures of patients' severity of illness become available. If outcomes, in addition to rates, are

---

*See also chapter 1 above.

monitored, hospital quality-assurance committees will doubtless be involved. In summary, monitoring and feedback seem certain to increase in the future. Both ideas on how to do this work and experience in implementing and improving such monitoring are necessary.

REFERENCES

1. Hampton, J.R. The end of clinical freedom. *Br Med J* 287:1237–48 (1983).
2. Luft, H.S. and Arno, P. Impact of increasing physician supply: A scenario for the future. *Health Affairs* 5:31–46 (1986).
3. Kralewski, J.E., Dowd, B., Feldman, R., and Shapiro, J. The physician rebellion. *N Eng J Med* 316:339–42 (1987).
4. Reinhardt, U.E. Resource allocation in health care: the allocation of lifestyles to providers. *Milbank Mem Fund Q.* 65:153–76 (1987).
5. Roch, D.J., Evans, R.G., and Pascoe, D.W. *Manitoba and Medicare—1971 to the Present.* Dept. of Research, Manitoba Health (1985).
6. Perrin, J.M., and Valvona, J. Does physician supply affect quality of care? *Health Affairs* 5:63–72 (1986).
7. Roos, N.P., Montgomery, P., and Roos, L.L. Health care utilization for the very elderly in the years prior to death. *Milbank Mem Fund Q* 65:231–54 (1987).
8. Manning, W.G., Leibowitz, A., Goldberg, G.A., et al. A controlled trial of the effect of a prepaid group practice on use of services. *N Eng J Med* 310:1505–10 (1984).
9. Stano, M. A further analysis of the "variations in practice style" phenomenon. *Inquiry* 23:176–82 (1986).
10. Roos, L.L., and Cageorge, S.M. Innovation, centralization, and growth: Coronary artery bypass graft surgery in Manitoba. Manuscript (1987).
11. Roos, L.L., Roos, N.P., Cageorge, S.M., and Nicol, J.P. How good are the data? Reliability of one health care data bank. *Med Care* 20:266–76 (1982).
12. Caper, P. The epidemiologic surveillance of medical care. *Am J Pub Hlth* 77:669–70 (1986).
13. Iglehart, J.K. Health policy report: Early experience with prospective payment of hospitals. *N Eng J Med* 314:1460–64 (1986).
14. Freeman, J.L., Fetter, R.B., and Newbold, R.C. Hospital utilization before and after the implementation of DRGs for hospital payment: U.S., 1979 to 1984. Journal Mgmt Med 1:309–23 (1987).
15. Mitchell, J.B. Physician DRGs. *N Eng J Med* 313:670–75 (1985).
16. Lichtenstein, J.L., Schneider, K.C., Freeman, J.L., et al. Ambulatory visit groups: an outpatient classification system. J Ambulatory Care Mgmt (forthcoming 88).
17. McMahon, L.F., and Newbold, R. Variation in resource use within diagnosis-related groups: The effect of severity of illness and physician practice. *Med Care* 24:388–97 (1986).

18. Worthman, L.G., and Cretin, S. *Review of the Literature on Diagnosis-Related Groups.* Rand N-2492-HCFA. Santa Monica, Cal.: Rand Corporation (1986).
19. Fetter, R.B. DRG refinement with diagnostic-specific co-morbidities and complications: A synthesis of current approaches to patient classification. Grant application to HCFA, November 4, 1986.
20. Roos, N.P. Differential use of outpatient surgery by hospitals and physicians: What are the potential savings? Manuscript (1987).
21. Horn, S.D. Misclassification problems in diagnosis-related groups: Cystic fibrosis as an example. *N Eng J Med* 314:484–87 (1986).
22. Thomas, J.W., Ashcraft, M.L.S., and Zimmerman, J. *An Evaluation of Alternative Severity-of-Illness Measures for Use by University Hospitals.* Dept. of Health Services Management and Policy, School of Public Health, University of Michigan, Technical Report (1986).
23. Wennberg, J.E., McPherson, K., and Caper, P. Will payment based on diagnosis-related groups control hospital costs? *N Eng J Med* 311:295–300 (1984).
24. Wennberg, J.E. Dealing with medical practice variations: A proposal for action. *Health Affairs* 3:6–32 (1984).
25. Pasley, B., Vernon, P., Gibson, G., et al. Variations in elderly hospital and surgical discharge rates, New York State. *Am J Pub Hlth* 77:679–84 (1987).
26. Wennberg, J.E., and Fowler, F.J. A test of consumer contributions to small-area variations in health care delivery. *J Maine Med Assoc* 68:275–79 (1977).
27. Roos, N.P., and Roos, L.L. High and low surgical rates: Risk factors for area residents. *Am J Pub Hlth* 71:591–600 (1981).
28. Roos, N.P., and Roos, L.L. Surgical rate variations: Do they reflect the health or socioeconomic characteristics of the population? *Med Care* 20:945–58 (1982).
29. Clark, J.L., and Hamilton, R.A. A primer on small-area analysis. *Michigan Hospitals* 22:37–47 (1986).
30. Roos, N.P., and Lyttle, D. The centralization of operations and access to treatment: Total hip replacement in Manitoba. *Am J Pub Hlth* 75:130–33 (1985).
31. American Medical Association. *Confronting Regional Variations: The Maine Approach.* Chicago: American Medical Association (1986).
32. Caper, J.D., and Spitzer, M. In defense of small-area analysis. *Health Affairs* 4:115–19 (1985).
33. Roos, L.L. Supply, workload, and utilization: A population-based analysis of surgery. *Am J Pub Hlth* 73:414–21 (1983).
34. Roos, L.L., Cageorge, S.M., Roos, N.P., and Danziger, R.G. Centralization, certification, and monitoring: Readmissions and complications after surgery. *Med Care* 24:1044–66 (1986).
35. Wennberg, J.E., Roos, N.P., Sola, L., et al. Use of claims-data systems to evaluate health care outcomes: Mortality and reoperation following prostatectomy. *JAMA* 257:933–36 (1987).

36. Roos, N.P., and Danzinger, R.G. Assessing surgical risks in a population: Patient histories before and after cholecystectomy. *Soc Sci and Med* 22:571–78 (1986).
37. Roos, N.P., Henteleff, P.D., and Roos, L.L. A new audit procedure applied to an old question: Is T & A justified? *Med Care* 15:1–18 (1977).
38. Roos, L.L. Alternative designs to study outcomes: The tonsillectomy case. *Med Care* 17:1069–87 (1979).
39. Abrams, H.B., Detsky, A.S., Roos, L.L., and Wajda, A. Is there a role for surgery in the acute management of infective endocarditis? A decision analysis and medical claims data base approach. Manuscript (1987).
40. Roos, N.P., Wennberg, J.E., and McPherson, K. Using DRGs for studying variations in hospital admission patterns. Paper presented at Conference on the Management of Financing of Hospital Services, London, England, December 1986. Health Care Fin Rev (forthcoming 88).
41. Pauker, S.G., and Kassirer, J.P. Decision analysis. *N Eng J Med* 316:250–58 (1987).
42. Sox, H.C. Decision analysis: A basic clinical skill. *N Eng J Med* 316:271–72 (1987).
43. Eisenman, B. *What Are My Chances?* Philadelphia: W.B. Saunders Co. (1980).
44. Showstack, J.A., Rosenfeld, K.E., Garnick, D.W., et al. Association of volume with outcome of coronary artery bypass graft surgery: Scheduled versus nonscheduled operations. *JAMA* 257:785–89 (1987).
45. Yeaton, W.H., and Wortman, P.M. The evaluation of coronary artery bypass graft surgery using data synthesis techniques. *Int J Tech Assess Health Care* 1:125–40 (1985).
46. Merrick, N.J., Brook, R.H., Fink, A., and Solomon, D.H. Use of carotid endarterectomy in five California Veterans Administration medical centers. *JAMA* 256:2531–35 (1986).
47. Plum, F. Extracranial-intracranial arterial bypass and cerebral vascular disease. *N Eng J Med* 313:1221–23 (1985).
48. Newcomer, R., Wood, J., and Sankar, A. Medicare prospective payment: Anticipated effects on hospitals, other community services, and families. *J Health Politics, Policy, and Law* 10:275–82 (1985).
49. Roos, L.L., Cageorge, S.M., Austen, E., and Lohr, K.N. Using computers to identify complications after surgery. *Am J Pub Hlth* 75:1288–95 (1985).
50. Luft, H.S., Bunker, J.P., and Enthoven, A.C. Should operations be regionalized? The empirical relation between surgical volume and mortality. *N Eng J Med* 301:1364–69 (1979).
51. Ware, J.E. Monitoring and evaluating health services. *Med Care* 23:705–9 (1985).
52. Hornbrook, M.C. Techniques for assessing hospital case mix. *Ann Rev Pub Hlth* 6:295–324 (1985).
53. Blumberg, M.S. Risk-adjusting health care outcomes: A methodologic review. *Med Care Rev* 43:351–93 (1986).
54. Mosteller, F., Gilbert, J.P., and McPeek, B. Reporting standards and research strategies for controlled trials. *Con Clin Trials* 1:37–58 (1980).

55. Mossey, J.M., and Roos, L.L. Using insurance claims to measure health status: The illness scale. *J Chron Dis* 40:41–49 (1987).
56. Wennberg, J.E. An experiment to improve the quality of care in hospitals: A proposal to the National Center for Health Services Research. Hanover, N.H.: Department of Community and Family Medicine, Dartmouth Medical School (1986).
57. Dyck, F.J., Murphy, F.A., Murphy, J.K., et al. Effect of surveillance on the number of hysterectomies in the province of Saskatchewan. *N Eng J Med* 286:1326–28 (1977).
58. McAfee, R.E. The hospital "surgical signature": A quality-assessment tool. *JAMA* 257:972 (1987).
59. Hannah, W.J. Indications for cesarean section: Final statement of the panel of the National Consensus Conference on aspects of cesarean birth. *Can Med Assoc J* 134:1348–52 (1986).
60. Lomas, L., and Enkin, M. Variations in operative delivery rates. *In:* Enkin, M., Chalmers, I., and Kerise, M., eds., *Effective Care in Pregnancy and Childbirth.* London: Oxford University Press (1987).
61. McCarthy, E.G., Finkel, M.L., and Ruchlin, H.S. *Second-Opinion Elective Surgery.* Boston, Mass.: Auburn House Publishing Co. (1981).
62. Wagner, D.P., Knaus, W.A., and Draper, E.A. The case for adjusting hospital rates for severity of illness. *Health Affairs* 5:148–53 (1986).

Index

Abdominal aortic aneurysm, 155
Abdominal surgery, 14
Abrams, H. L., 147
ACS (American College of Surgeons), 30, 31, 36; critical of GMENAC report, 33
Adams, D. F., 147
Adenoidectomy: decline of incidence of, 45, 53; NIH evaluation of procedures for, 164
Admissions, 7; inappropriate, 137; surgical, 107–20. See also DHA (discretion in hospital admissions) measure
Ambulatory surgery. See Surgery, ambulatory
Ambulatory surgery center (ASC), 1, 7, 138
Ambulatory surgery utilization (ASU) measure, 112–13, 116, 120
American College of Surgeons. See ACS
American Medical Association, 166
American Surgical Association (ASA), 30
American Telephone and Telegraph Company, 71
Anesthesiology, 97; advances in, 125, 162
Aneurysm, abdominal aortic, 155
Angina pectoris, 50, 58, 91; coronary artery disease and, 83; hospitalization for, 115; social aspects of incidence of, 96
Angiography, 89, 94, 99
Angioplasty, 92, 99, 103; percutaneous, 94–95; transluminal percutaneous, 50
Anterior cruciate ligament syndrome, 51
Antibiotics: for benign prostatic obstruction, 94; for bladder ailments, 91
Antisepsis, 126
Antithrombotic drugs, 164
Appendectomy, 11, 44
Arteriography, 8, 41, 147
Artery disease. See Coronary artery disease
Arthrocentesis, 43
Arthroplasty, hip, 43
Arthroscopic surgery, 51
ASA (American Surgical Association), 30
ASC (ambulatory surgery center), 1, 7, 138
Asthma: hospitalization for acute, 160; hospitalization patterns for pediatric, 111
ASU (ambulatory surgery utilization) measure, 112–13, 116, 120
Atherosclerosis, coronary, 91; hospitalization patterns for, 107
Atherosclerotic occlusive brain disease, 167
Augusta, Me., 68, 69

Back problems, hospitalization for, 68, 69
Back surgery, 51; hospitalization patterns for, 111
Bane Committee Report, 30
Barer, M. L., 119
Barnes, B. A., 53
Barnsley, Janet M., 4
Bartholin's cyst, 91
Bayne-Jones Report, 30
Beta-blocking, 164
Biliary tract, disorders of, 107
Biopsy, breast, 58, 90, 93, 101
Bladder: changes in, 87–88; extrophy of, 82

191

Bladder neck obstruction, 88, 91, 94
Blide, L. A., 109
Blue Cross, FASC and, 127
Blue Shield, 66
Boston, Mass., 67, 84–85
Boston University, 85
Brain disease, 167
Breast biopsy, 58, 90, 93, 101
Breast cancer, 13, 82, 90, 161, 163; NIH evaluation of surgical procedures for, 164; OTA evaluation of surgical procedures for, 168; surgery for, 15; TOPPS ratios for, 101–2; treatment of, 93
Breast lumps, 90
British Columbia, 116
Bronchitis, 58; ambulatory treatment of, 63; hospitalization patterns for pediatric, 111
Brookline, Mass., 85
Brunswick, Me., 70
Bulletin of the American College of Surgeons, 33
Bunker, J. P., 13
Bypass surgery. *See* Coronary artery bypass surgery

Calais, Me., 68
California, Medicaid in, 144
Cambridge, Mass., 85
Canada: health care expenditures in, 16; hospital beds in, 15; hospital costs in, 117; national health insurance of, 19–20; surgeon population of, 15; surgery in, 12–20, 44, 110. *See also* British Columbia; Manitoba; Ontario; Saskatchewan
Cancer, 184; breast (*see* Breast cancer); cervical, 13; cholecystectomy and, 11; and NIH research, 163–64; nonmetastic prostatic, 164; prostatic, 15; uterine, 13
Candidate cohort, TOPPS, 90–92, 180
Caper, P., 44, 117, 179

Carcinoma. *See* Cancer
Cardiac surgery, 97, 98. *See also* Coronary artery bypass surgery
Cardiology, 97
Cardiopulmonary disease, 184. *See also* Heart failure, congestive; Myocardial infarction
Cardiovascular disease, 164
Cardiovascular surgeons, 27; surplus of, 32
Cardiovascular surgery, 27, 182; effect of new technology on, 34. *See also* Coronary artery bypass surgery
Carotid disease, asymptomatic, 168
Cataract surgery. *See* Lens extraction
Catheterization: for benign prostatic obstruction, 94; for bladder ailments, 91; cardiac, 8, 41, 94, 103, 145–53
Cesarean section, 15, 18, 91, 160–61; cost of, 47–49; cost of vs. vaginal delivery, 49; incidence of, 47–49; NIH evaluation of surgical procedures for, 164; in Ontario, 19–20; proliferation of, 45; regional variations in incidence of, 47; repeat, 185; TOPPS ratios for, 102
Chassin, M. R., 42
Chemotherapy, 93, 102
Chest pain, 92; hospitalization patterns for, 111. *See also* Angina pectoris
Children: hospitalization of, 111, 160; tonsillectomy and, 54
Cholecystectomy, 4, 13–15, 18, 44, 49–50, 180; for asymptomatic gallstones, 19; and cancer, 11; complications from, 181; costs of, 43; regional variations in incidence of, 50; in Sweden, 12–13; in women, 13
Cholera, 83
Clinics, walk-in, 1
Colon, surgery on, 23
Commission on Professional and

Hospital Activities (CPHA), 145–46
Commonwealth Fund, 73, 75
Co-morbidity, 179
Connell, F. A., 109
Consumerism, "unnecessary" surgery and, 34
Cooperative Studies Program, VA, 168
Copayment, 108
Coronary artery bypass surgery, 43, 50–51, 92, 97, 99, 180, 181; alternatives to, 50; angina pectoris as indication for, 83; costs of, 50–51; and Council on Health Care Technology, 170; discretionary/nondiscretionary status of, 12; elderly and, 47; for Medicare beneficiaries, 161; for myocardial infarction, 160; myocardial infarction following, 182; NIH evaluation of surgical procedures for, 164; proliferation of, 45, 50
Coronary artery disease, 82, 91, 94; angina pectoris and, 83; chronic, 103
Coronary atherosclerosis, 91
Coronary disease, causes of, 91–92
Coronary heart disease: and hospital "team" concept, 97; TOPPS ratios for, 103
Coronary insufficiency, chronic, 91
Coronary syndrome, intermediate, 91
Corporations, employee health and, 71, 76
Council on Health Care Technology, 170, 172
CPHA (Commission on Professional and Hospital Activities), 145–46
C-section. See Cesarean section
Curettage. See Dilation and curettage
Cyclosporine, 168
Cystic fibrosis, 54
Cystoscopy, 58, 67–68; as treatment for benign prostatic obstruction, 94
Czechoslovakia, 18

D&C. See Dilation and curettage
Death. See Mortality
Defibrillator, implantable, 169
Denmark, 18
Dental extractions, hospitalization for, 58, 69, 111
Dental implants, NIH evaluation of, 164
DHA (discretion in hospital admissions) measure, 111–13, 116, 120
Diabetes, 114; and distal gangrene, 99; hospitalization for, 109, 115; juvenile, 86
Diagnosis-related groups. See DRGs
Digitalis, 86
Dilation and curettage, 86, 91
Discharge abstracts, 183
Discretion in hospital admissions. See DHA
Doctors. See Physicians; Surgeons
Draper, E. A., 185
DRGs (diagnosis-related groups), 1, 20, 44, 64, 68, 69, 78, 109, 111–12, 136, 178–79, 184
Drugs, 9; antithrombotic, 164; FDA and, 165
Dyck, F. J., 185
Dysrhythmia, 92, 146
Dysuria, 91

Ear, middle, 97
Ear-nose-throat surgery. See ENT surgery
EC-IC (extracranial-intracranial) arterial bypass surgery, 167, 181
Eimerl, T. S., 12, 13
Eisenberg, J. M., 109
Eisenman, B., 181
Elderly, hospitalization and, 107–8, 113–14, 116, 160, 176. See also Medicaid; Medicare
Electrocardiography, 166
Employers, health care and, 1–2, 9

Endarterectomy, carotid, 167–68
Endoscopy: advances in, 162; diagnostic upper gastrointestinal, 43
England: health care expenditures in, 16; hospital beds in, 15; surgeon population of, 15; surgery in, 12–18, 20, 44. See also Liverpool, Eng.; Scotland; United Kingdom; Wales
ENT (ear-nose-throat): surgeons, surplus of, 32; surgery, 26
Epidemiology, clinical, 74, 75
Epstein, A., 16, 181
Ermann, Dan, 7, 183
Ethics, 9, 168
Europe, surgery in, 18
Evans, R. G., 109
Ewing Report, 30
Excision, lens. See Lens extraction
Extended-care facilities, 184
Extracranial-intracranial (EC-IC) arterial bypass surgery, 167, 181
Extractions, dental, hospitalization for, 58, 69, 111
Extrophy, of bladder, 82
Eye surgery, 14. See also Lens extraction

Fallot, Tetralogy of, 82
Farr, William, 70
FASCs (freestanding ambulatory surgery centers), 127–34, 161; and Medicare, 162
FDA (Food and Drug Administration), 163, 165
Femur, fracture of, 85, 86
Foltz, A., 42
Food and Drug Administration (FDA), 163, 165
Forearm fracture, ambulatory treatment of, 63
France, 13
Fraser, D. B., 147
Free-Standing Ambulatory Surgery Association, 132
Freestanding ambulatory surgery centers. See FASCs

Gallbladder, surgery on, 13, 18. See also Cholecystectomy
Gallbadder disease, 15, 180; in women, 13
Gallstones, 50, 83, 180; asymptomatic, 4, 11, 19, 50
Gangrene, distal, 99
Gastroenteritis, 58
Gastrointestinal endoscopy, diagnostic upper, 43
General surgeons, 24; surplus of, 32
Genital tract, malignant diseases of, 15
Gilbert, J. P., 184
Gittelsohn, A. M., 43, 72, 81, 87, 127
Glover, J. A., 43
GMENAC (Graduate Medical Education National Advisory Committee), 32–33
Government, assessment of surgical procedures by, 159–72
Gracie, W. A., 21
Graduate Medical Education National Advisory Committee (GMENAC), 32–33
Gynecologic surgery, 14, 45; precluded by second opinion, 4. See also Obstetric-gynecolgoic surgery

Hampton, J. R., 175
Hanken, M. A., 109
Hanley, Daniel, 72
Harvard University, 85
Haug, James, 31
Hawthorne effect, 185
HCFA (Health Care Financing Administration), 166, 167
Health care, 1–10; costs of, 9, 176–79; employers and, 1–2, 9; future of, 9; insurers and, 2, 9; surgery and delivery of, 125–43
Health Care Financing Administration (HCFA), 75, 166, 167
Health insurance, 19–20
Health maintenance organizations (HMOs), 1, 34, 42, 62, 109,

134–37, 161, 177
Health Professions Educational Assistance Act, 30, 32
Health Promotion and Disease Prevention Amendments of 1984, 167, 170
Heart, artificial, 165, 168
Heart disease: chronic ischemic, 91; nonsurgical treatment of, 50. *See also* Angina pectoris; Atherosclerosis, coronary; Cardiopulmonary disease; Cardiovascular disease; Coronary artery disease; Coronary disease; Coronary heart disease; Heart failure; Myocardial infarction
Heart failure, 86, 92, 146; congestive, 184
Heart transplantation, 166
Heart valves, 165
Hebel, J. R., 157
Hemorrhoidectomy, 12, 13, 44, 86–87
Hemorrhoids: injection of, 43; patient self-treatment of, 93
Hernia: inguinal, 43, 61; surgery on, 31, 44
Herniated intervertebral disc disease, 12
Herniorrhaphy, inguinal, 13, 14, 85, 86
Hip: arthroplasty of, 43; fracture of, 61, 63; replacement of, 88, 97, 98, 180
Hip joint, NIH evaluation of surgical procedures for replacement of, 164
Hlatky, M., 42
HMOs. *See* Health maintenance organizations
Home health care, 1
Hormone therapy, 83
Hospital industry, 59
Hospitalization, 2–3; and admission, 7; arbitrariness of, 58–78; of elderly, 107–8, 113–14, 116, 176; patient-harmful, 114; physician-discretionary, 107–20; quality of care during, 144–57; regionalization and, 144–57. *See also* Surgery, ambulatory
Hospitals: indisposition of to accept certain types of patient, 99; and reputation factor, 7; TOPPS ratios for, 103–4. *See also* Hospitalization
Hughes, E.F.X., 31
Hunt, Sandra S., 8
Hyperplasia, prostatic, 58, 60–61
Hypertension, 82; hospitalization for, 115
Hyperthyroidism, 12
Hypertrophy: prostatic, 53, 70, 88, 91; of tonsil, 58, 61
Hysterectomy, 15, 18, 44, 45, 61, 90–91; in Canada, 13; complications from, 181; cost of, 53, 63; and elderly, 47; in New England, 12, 13; for noncancerous conditions, 4, 11, 60; nonsurgical alternatives to, 86; regional incidence of, 52–53; in Saskatchewan, 12; TOPPS ratios for, 102; unnecessary, 3; vaginal bleeding as indication for, 83

ICDA (International Classification of Disease Adapted), 12
Incarceration, hernial, 11
Incontinence, 91
Indarterectomy, carotid, 181
Infection: hospital-acquired, 114, 126, 132, 154, 161; nosocomial, 161
Institute of Medicine (IOM), 169–70, 172
Insulin, 86
Insurers: health care and, 2, 9, 117; and ambulatory surgery, 162
Intensive care, 97
Intermediate coronary syndrome, 91
International Classification of Disease Adapted (ICDA), 12
Intervertebral cartilage, excision of, 51
Intervertebral disc, excision of, 23

Invasion, vascular, 94
IOM (Institute of Medicine), 169–70, 172
Iowa, 61; medical costs-containment program in, 72
Ischemic heart disease, chronic, 91
Ischemic stroke, arterial bypass surgery for, 167

Jaundice, 11
John A. Hartford Foundation, 75
Joint replacement, 168
Jones, L. W., 30

Kaiser-Permanente Medical Care Program, 109, 126, 171
Keratometers, intraoperative, 161
Kidney transplant, 160
Knaus, W. A., 185
Knee replacement, 180
Knee surgery, 51–52; hospitalization patterns for, 111
Knickman, J., 42
Kralewski, J. E., 176

Laser therapy, 8, 41, 162
Lee, R. I., 30
Lenses, intraocular, 52, 164, 165
Lens extraction, 11, 14, 16, 17, 52, 160; on ambulatory basis, 161–62; cost of, 43, 52; elderly and, 47; extracapsular, 161; improvements in technology of, 161; incidence of, 52; and insertion of intraocular lens, 165; proliferation of, 45
Leukoplakia, 91
Lewis, C. E., 30
Lewis, C. L., 81
Lewiston, Me., 68
Life expectancy, 1
Lister, Joseph, 126
Lithotripsy, extracorporeal shockwave, 168
Liverpool, Eng., 12–13
Liver transplantation, 164

Logan, R.F.L., 12, 13
Lomas, J., 119
Luft, Harold S., 8
Lumpectomy, 93
Lumps, breast, 90
Lung disease, hospitalization for chronic obstructive, 117
Lyme disease, 83
Lymph node, dissection of, 93

McAfee, R. E., 185
McPeek, B., 184
McPherson, K., 16–17, 44, 117, 179
Magnetic resonance, nuclear, 8
Maine: corporate input in hospitalization patterns in, 76–77; cystoscopic services in, 67–68; decline of incidence of tonsillectomy in, 88; hospitalization in, 67–69; incidence of hysterectomy in, 61–63; incidence of prostatectomy in, 73; incidence of surgery in, 86; incidence of tonsillectomy in, 62
Maine Health Information Center, 71, 77
Maine Medical Assessment Program, 184, 185
Maine Medical Association, 72–73, 75
Malpractice, hospital, 154, 156
Managed care, 1
Manitoba, Can.: hospitalization patterns in, 108–16; nursing homes of, 116; surgery in, 61, 180
Manitoba Health Services Commission, 115
Maryland Blue Cross, 139
Massachusetts, 44, 96. See also Boston, Mass.
Massachusetts Health Data Consortium, 97
Massachusetts Institute of Technology (MIT), 85
Mastectomy, 85, 93, 101; in Canada, 13
Mediastinoscopy, 43

Medicaid, 66, 77; in California, 144
Medical Applications of Research, Office of, 164
Medical schools, 31–34
Medicare, 54, 66, 117, 126; and ambulatory surgery, 138; and arterial bypass surgery for ischemic stroke, 167; and carotid endarterectomy, 167–68; and cataract surgery, 52; and coronary artery bypass surgery, 161; and DRGs, 178–79; and freestanding ambulatory surgery centers, 162; and heart transplantation, 166; in Manitoba, 109; and OHTA, 167; and ProPac, 169; and prospective payment system, 181; statistical potential of, 71. See also HCFA (Health Care Financing Administration)
Medicine: academic, 74–75; "defensive," 59, 78
Meniscectomy, 52
Menopause, 83, 86; surgical treatment of symptoms of, 58
Menstrual disorders, hysterectomy to correct, 53
Microscopes, surgical, 161
Microsurgery, 51, 125
Middle ear, reconstruction of, 97
Milbank Memorial Fund, 75
Mindell, W. R., 14
MIT (Massachusetts Institute of Technology), 85
Mobil Oil Company, 139
Molars, removal of third, 164
Moore, F. D., 6, 33, 34, 179, 180
Morrisville, Vt., 72
Mortality: cancer and, 13; after cardiac catheterization, 145–53; and gallbladder disease, 13
Moscovice, I. S., 109
Mosteller, F., 184
Mountin-Pennel-Berger forecast, 30
Multihospital systems, 1, 7, 134, 136–37
Myocardial infarction, 63; acute, 91, 92, 94, 99, 154, 184; after coronary artery bypass surgery, 182; hospitalization for, 160–61; old, 91

National Academy of Sciences, 169–70
National Advisory Council on Health Care Technology Assessments, 167
National Cancer Institute, 163
National Center for Health Care Technology, 75
National Center for Health Services Research, 75
National Center for Health Services Research and Health Care Technology Assessment (NCHSR), 165, 167
National Center for Health Statistics (NCHS), 22, 45
National Heart, Lung, and Blood Institute, 163–64
National Institutes of Health (NIH), 163–64
NCHS (National Center for Health Statistics), 22, 45
NCHSR (National Center for Health Services Research and Health Care Technology Assessment), 165, 167
Neck surgery, 111
Netherlands, 18
Neurosurgeons, 28; surplus, 32
Neurosurgery, 14, 23, 28; effect of new technology on, 34
Newborn, congenital anomalies in, 99
New England, 12–13, 17, 44. See also Maine; Massachusetts; Vermont
New Haven, Conn., 67, 84–85
Nightingale, Florence, 70
NIH (National Institutes of Health), 163–64
Nocturia, 91
North America, surgery in, 18
Norway: lens extraction in, 62; surgery in, 17, 18, 44

Nuclear magnetic resonance, 8, 41
Nursing homes, 184; of Manitoba, 116

Obesity, surgical treatment of morbid, 164
Obstetric-gynecologic surgeons, 32
Obstetric-gynecologic surgery, 24–25. *See also* Gynecologic surgery
Obstetrician-gynecologists, 24–25
Office of Health Technology Assessment (OHTA), 165–68, 171
Office of Medical Applications of Research, 164
Office of Technology Assessment (OTA), 168, 169
OHTA (Office of Health Technology Assessment), 165–68, 171
Omnibus Budget Reconciliation Act of 1980, 138, 162
Ontario, Can.: hospitalization patterns in, 109; surgery in, 18
Ophthalmic centers, 130
Ophthalmologic surgeons, 26; surplus of, 32
Ophthalmologic surgery, 26; effect of new technology on, 34; unnecessary, 3
Ophthalmologists, and lens-extraction, 52
Ophthalmology: FDA and, 165; technological advances in, 161
Orthopedic surgeons, 25; surplus of, 32
Orthopedic surgery, 14, 23, 25, 51; effect of new technology on, 34; precluded by second opinion, 4; unnecessary, 3
OTA (Office of Technology Assessment), 168, 169
Otolaryngologic surgery, 14
Otorhinolaryngology. *See* ENT (ear-nose-throat) surgery
Outcomes, 144–57, 181–83, 185
Outpatients. *See* Surgery, ambulatory

Pacemakers, implantable, 165; Pro-Pac and, 169
PAS (Professional Activity Studies), 145
Pascoe, D. W., 109
PDML (Physician Distribution and Medical Licensure), 23
Pearson, R.J.C., 13
Peer-review organizations (PROs), 159, 169
Penile prosthesis, 169
Peptic ulcer, 111
Percutaneous angioplasty, 94–95; transluminal, 50
Perinatal mortality rate (PMR), 18
Perrin, J. M., 176
Phoenix, Ariz., 127
PHS (physician hospitalization style) measure, 113–15
Physician Distribution and Medical Licensure (PDML), 23
Physician hospitalization style (PHS) measure, 113–15
Physicians. *See* ENT (ear-nose-throat) surgeons; General surgeons; Neurosurgeons; Obstetric-gynecologic surgeons; Obstetrician-gynecologists; Ophthalmologic surgeons; Ophthalmologists; Orthopedic surgeons; Plastic surgeons; Surgeons
Pittsburgh, Pa., 116
Plant, J.C.D., 13
Plastic surgeons, 32
Plastic surgery, 23
PMR (perinatal mortality rate), 18
Pneumonectomy, 11
Pneumonia, pediatric, 111, 117
Portland, Me., 68
Portland, Ore., 127
PPOs (preferred provider organizations), 1, 134–36, 144, 177
Practice style, 58–59, 61–63, 70, 81–83, 87, 97, 108–10, 115, 177. *See also* PHS (physician hospitalization style) measure
Preadmission certification, 1
Preferred provider organizations

(PPOs), 1, 134–36, 144, 177
President's Commission on the Health Needs of the Nation, 30
Professional Activity Studies (PAS), 145
Professional standards review organizations (PSROs), 159
ProPac (Prospective Payment Commission), 169
PROs (peer-review organizations), 159, 169
Prospective Payment Commission (ProPac), 169
Prospective rate setting, 1
Prostate: benign obstruction of, 93–94; cancer of, 15; hyperplasia of, 58, 60–61; hypertrophy of, 53, 70; nonmetastic cancer of, 164; surgery on, 53
Prostatectomy, 15, 43, 44, 61, 91; for benign hyperplasia of prostate, 60–61; complications from, 181; federal government and, 75; limitations of, 87–88; open, 94; for prostatic hypertrophy, 70; risks of, 181; second, 70; in Sweden, 12–13; TOPPS ratios for, 102; transurethral, 91, 94, 102
Prosthesis: joint, 169; penile, 169
Providence, R.I., 127
PSROs (professional standards review organizations), 159
Pyelonephritis, ascending, 88

Quadrantectomy, 93

Radiation therapy, 93, 102
Radiology, 97
Rand Health Insurance Experiment, 108, 134
Ranshoff, D. F., 21
Rates, prospective, 1
Readmissions, 181–82, 185
Rectal surgery, 23
Referral effect, 7, 183
Regionalization of hospital care, 7–8, 144–57
Reimbursement, 7, 8, 42, 138–39. *See also* Third-party payers
Reinhardt, U. E., 176
Renal failure, 146
Residency, surgical, 32–33
Respiratory distress syndrome, 160
Robert Wood Johnson Foundation, 75
Roch, D. J., 109
Roemer hypothesis, 42
Roos, L. L., 7, 18, 180
Roos, N. P., 7, 18, 44, 62, 117, 120, 180
Rosenblatt, R. A., 109
Ross-Loos Health Plan, 134
Ruby, Gloria, 9
Rumford, Me., 67–68
Rutkow, I. M., 4, 14, 175

San Francisco, Calif., 160
Saskatchewan: hysterectomy in, 62, 114, 185; surgery in, 12
SAV (small-area variation) method, 5–6, 81–88, 93–96, 179–80
Scitovsky, A. A., 8, 160
Scotland, 18
Second opinions, 3–4, 109, 137–38, 185; mandatory, 1
Sentinel effect, 138
Shock-wave lithotripsy, extracorporeal, 168
Showstack, J. A., 160
Sinusitis, 54
Sioux City, Ia., 126
Sisk, Jane E., 9
Sloan, F. A., 47, 160
Small-area variation. *See* SAV
Sodertalje, Sweden, 12–13
SOSSUS (*Study on Surgical Services for the United States*), 30–31
Spina bifida, 99
Spinal fusion, 51
SSCS (Survey of Specialized Clinical Services), 145
Stano, M., 177

Sterilization, surgical, 45, 58, 84; hysterectomy for purpose of, 53. *See also* Vasectomy
Stoddart, G. L., 119
Strangulation, hernial, 11
Stroke, ischemic. *See* Ischemic stroke
Strong, P. M., 16
Study on Surgical Services for the United States (SOSSUS), 30–31
Support systems, 9
Surgeons: general (*see* General surgeons); indisposition of to accept certain cases, 99; nonboard certified, 34; surplus of, 4, 32–36, 175–77; as teachers, 35. *See also* ENT (ear-nose-throat) surgeons; Neurosurgeons; Obstetric-gynecologic surgeons; Ophthalmologic surgeons; Orthopedic surgeons; Plastic surgeons
surgeons
Surgery, 3–4; age as a factor in, 45–47; ambulatory, 23, 110, 112–13, 126–34, 161–62, 177, 180, 183 (*see also* FASCs); in armed forces, 12; and burn victims, 99; on children, 53–54; commonest types of, 4, 29; cost of, 3, 11–20, 41–54; day (*see* Surgery, ambulatory); demographic aspects of, 5; in developed nations, 4, 11–20; and "difficult" cases, 99; discretionary, 11–13; and distal gangrene, 99; elective, 3; evaluation of care relative to, 6, 80–104; future of, 35, 175–86; general, 24; government and, 5, 9, 159–72; health care delivery and, 125–43; in-and-out (*see* Surgery, ambulatory); incidence of, 45–55; NIH evaluation of, 163–64; nondiscretionary, 11–12, 13, 18; open heart, 166; outpatient (*see* Surgery, ambulatory); and Parkinson's Law, 30; payment for (*see* Reimbursement); as profession, 4; regional variation in cost of, 5; regional variations in incidence of, 5, 58–79; regional variations in procedures of, 7–8, 41–57; and safety, 6; and skill, 8; survival of, 7–8; unnecessary, 3–5, 7, 11, 19, 22, 34, 43–44, 54, 127, 135–36, 139, 175. *See also* individual procedures (e.g., catheterization) *and specializations* (e.g., cholecystectomy)
Surgical centers, ambulatory, 1
Surgicenters, 127
Survey of Specialized Clinical Services (SSCS), 145
Sweden, 12–13, 18
Syracuse, N.Y., 110

Technology, 8–9; government and, 9; medical, 44, 70, 162–72; proliferation of, 8; ultrasound, 8, 41
Tetralogy of Fallot, 82
Third-party payers, 8, 154–56, 159; and ambulatory surgery, 162; and surgical innovations, 163
Thoracic surgeons, 32
Thoracic surgery, 27; effect of new technology on, 34
Thyroidectomy, 12
Ticks, 83
Tomography, 8; computerized, 41
Tonsil, hypertrophy of, 58, 61
Tonsilitis, 53–54
Tonsillectomy, 11, 14, 18, 44, 85; decline in incidence of, 45, 53–54, 88; in England, 43; hospitalization patterns for, 107, 111; for hypertrophy of tonsil, 61; in New England, 13; NIH evaluation of surgical procedures for, 164; in Saskatchewan, 12; unnecessary, 3
TOPPS (treatment options and practice profiles), 89–104
Traction, 86
Treatment options and practice pro-

files (TOPPS), 89–104
Tubal interruptions, hospitalization patterns for, 111
Tubal sterilization. *See* Sterilization, surgical
Tufts University, 85
Typhus, 83

Ulcer, peptic, 107, 111
Ultrasound technology, 8, 41; ultrasonography, 98
United Kingdom: health care expenditures in, 16; surgery in, 12, 20. *See also* England; Scotland; Wales
Uppsala, Sweden, 13
Ureterovesical reflux, 88
Urologic surgeons, 26; surplus of, 32
Urologic surgery, 26
Urology, ambulatory surgery and, 127
Uropathy, obstructive, 91
Uterus, fibroids of, 82

VA (Veterans Administration), 163, 168, 171
Vaginal bleeding, 83–84; manifold treatment options for, 86
Valvona, J., 47, 160, 176

Varicose veins, 11–13
Vasectomy, 84
Vascular surgery, 34
Vayda, E., 4, 13, 14
Vermont, 61, 62, 72, 116
Vermont Medical Society, 72
Vertebral surgery, 45
Veterans Administration (VA), 163, 168, 171
Viscoelastic substances, 161

Wagner, D. P., 185
Wales: health care expenditures in, 16; hospital beds in, 15; surgeon population of, 15; surgery in, 13–18
Walk-in clinics, 1
Waterville, Me., 67–69
Wennberg, J. E., 5–6, 43, 44, 81, 87, 117, 127, 179, 184, 185
Williams, D. C., 31, 33
Women, surgical sterilization of, 45, 53, 84

X-rays, 126

Yale University, 84
Yale University Health Plan (YHP), 84

NO LONGER THE PROPERTY
OF THE
UNIVERSITY OF R.I. LIBRARY